THE ARTS OF BEAUTY

NEW YORK

The Ecco Press

1 WEST 30TH STREET

THE ARTS OF

Beauty

OR,

SECRETS OF A LADY'S TOILET.

WITH HINTS TO GENTLEMEN ON THE ART OF

Fascinating

BY

Madame Lola Montez

COUNTESS OF LANDSFELD

Published by The Ecco Press in 1978
1 West 30th Street, New York, New York   10001
Published simultaneously in Canada by
Penguin Books Canada Ltd.
Printed in the United States of America
The Ecco Press logo by Ahmed Yacoubi
Designed by Cynthia Krupat
Library of Congress Cataloging in Publication Data
Montez, Lola, 1818-1861.
The arts of beauty.   Includes index.
1. Beauty, Personal.   I. Title.
RA778.M75   1978   646.7   77-19081
ISBN 0-912-94652-0
ISBN 0-912-94653-9 (paperback)

TABLE

OF CONTENTS

HINTS TO GENTLEMEN
ON THE ART OF FASCINATING

INTRODUCTORY

REMARKS

*W*hen Aristotle was asked why everybody was so fond of beauty, he replied, "It is the question of a blind man." Socrates described it as "a short-lived tyranny;" and Theophrastus called it "a silent fraud." Most of these old philosophers spoke in great scorn and derision of the arts employed by the females of their time for the display and preservation of their beauty. And it would seem that the ladies of those days carried these arts to greater extremes than even our modern belles. Juvenal bitterly satirizes the women's faces as being "bedaubed and lacquered o'er." The Roman belles used chalk and paint in a most extravagant profusion, as we must infer from Martial, who tells us that "Fabula was afraid of the rain, on account of the chalk on her face; and Lobella of the sun, because of the *céruse* with which her face was painted; and the famous Poppæa, the first mistress, and afterwards the wife of Nero, made use of an unctuous paint, which hardened upon her face, and entirely changed the original features."

A history of all the arts which my sex have employed, since her creation, to set off and preserve her charms, would not only far exceed the limits of this volume, but it would be a tedious and useless book when written. I shall confine myself mainly to the *modern arts* which have fallen within my own observation during an experience which has extended to nearly all the courts and fashionable cities of the principal nations of the earth. The recipes which I shall give for the various cosmetics, washes, pastes, creams, powders, etc., are such as are in use among the fashionable belles of the various capitals of the Old World. I give them as *curiosities*, desiring that they may pass for what they are worth, and no more. If, however, a lady wishes to use such helps to beauty, I must advise her, by all means, to become *her own manufacturer*—not only as a matter of *economy*, but of *safety*—as many of the patent cosmetics have ruined the finest complexions, and induced diseases of the skin and of the nervous system, which have embittered the life, and prematurely ended the days of their victims. For a few shillings, and with a little pains, any lady can provide herself with a bountiful supply of all such things, composed of materials, which, at any rate, are harmless, and which are far superior to the expensive patent compounds which she buys of druggists. Some years ago, there was an amusing controversy and lawsuit in England about a famous lotion for "improving and beautifying the complexion." A Mr. Dickinson, a Mrs. Vincent, and a Mr. MacDonald, each claimed to be the inventor of the popular and profitable cosmetic, which sold for seven shillings and sixpence the pint bottle. The lawsuit disclosed both the materials and the cost of the compound, which were as follows:

One and a half ounce of bitter almonds . . 1½d.

Fifteen grains of corrosive sublimate . . . ½

One quart of water	0
Bottle	3
Cost of a quart	5d.

So that this fashionable lotion, which sold for seven shillings and sixpence a pint, cost only five pence a quart, being a profit of *seventeen hundred per cent*. . . . And it will be readily admitted that any lady who wished to treat her face to a dose of corrosive sublimate, could buy the ingredients and compound them herself, as easily as Mr. Dickinson and Mrs. Vincent. There was another famous cosmetic, called *Lignum's Lotion*, which was nothing more than a solution of sal-ammoniac in water, and cost three pence half-penny a quart, and it was sold for five shillings. This, like nearly all the patent preparations, was entirely useless, except to delude the vanity of my sex, and make money for its inventor.

It is to guard women against these monstrous impositions, and to save them from such needless and useless expenditures, that I have encumbered this work with so many *recipes*. They were, many of them, given me by celebrated beauties who used them themselves; and most of them were, originally, written in the French, Spanish, German, and Italian languages. In translating them, I am painfully impressed that I may have used many unprofessional terms, even if I have committed no worse blunders; but, if my meaning is intelligible, they may, I think, be relied upon as the safest and best preparations which a lady can employ in her toilet.

The Baroness de Staël confessed that she would exchange half her knowledge for personal charms, and there is not much doubt that most women of genius, to whom nature has denied the talismanic power of beauty, would consider it cheaply bought at that price. And let not man deride her sacrifice, and call it *vanity*, until he becomes himself so morally purified and intellectually elevated that he would prefer the society of an ugly woman of genius to that of a great and matchless beauty of less intellectual acquirements. All women know that it is *beauty*, rather than *genius*, which all generations of men have worshipped in our sex. Can it be wondered at, then, that so much of our attention should be directed to the means of developing and preserving our charms? When men speak of the *intellect* of woman, they speak critically, tamely, coldly; but when they come to speak of the *charms of a beautiful woman*, both their language and their eyes kindle with the glow of an enthusiasm, which shows them to be profoundly, if not, indeed, ridiculously in earnest. It is a part of our natural sagacity to perceive all this, and we should be enemies to ourselves if we did not employ every allowable art to become the goddesses of that adoration. Preach to the contrary as you may, there still stands the eternal fact, that the world has yet allowed no higher "mission" to woman, than to be *beautiful*. Taken in the best meaning of that word, it may be fairly questioned if there *is* any higher mission for woman on earth. But, whether there *is*, or *is not*, there is no such thing as making *female beauty* play a less part than it already does, in the *admiration of man* and in the *ambition of woman*. With great propriety, if it did not spoil the poetry, might we alter Mr. Pope's famous line on happiness, so as to make it read—

"O beauty! our being's end and aim."

My design in this volume is to discuss the various Arts employed by my sex in the pursuit of this paramount object of woman's life. I have aimed to make a *useful* as well as an *entertaining* and *amusing* book. The fortunes of life have given to my own experience, or observation, nearly all the materials of which it is composed. So, if the volume is of less importance than I have estimated, it must be charged to my want of *capacity*, and not to any lack of *information* on the subject of which it treats.

The *Hints to Gentlemen on the Art of Fascinating*, I am sure, will prove amusing to the ladies. And I shall be disappointed if it fails to be a useful and instructive lesson to the other gender. The men have been laughing, I know not how many thousands of years, at the *vanity* of women, and if the women have not been able to return the compliment, and laugh at the *vanity* on the other side of the house, it is only because they have been wanting in a proper knowledge of the bearded gender.

If my "Hints" shall prove to be a looking-glass in which the men can "see themselves as others see them," they will, I hope, not be unthankful for the favor I have done them. And if my own sex receives this book in the same spirit with which I have addressed myself to its subject, I shall be happy in the conviction that I have rendered my experience serviceable to them and honorable to myself.

Lola Montez

THE ARTS OF BEAUTY

CHAPTER I

FEMALE BEAUTY

"*Look upon this face,*
Examine every feature and proportion,
And you with me must grant this rare piece finish'd.
Nature, despairing e'er to make the like,
Brake suddenly the mould in which 'twas fashion'd;
Yet, to increase your pity, and call on
Your justice with severity, this fair outside
Was but the cover of a fairer mind."

Massinger's *Parliament of Love*.

*I*t is a most difficult task to fix upon any general and satisfactory standard of female beauty, since forms and qualities the most opposite and contradictory are looked upon by different nations, and by different individuals, as the perfection of beauty. Some will have it that a beautiful woman must be *fair*, while others conceive nothing but brunettes to be handsome. A Chinese belle must be fat, have small eyes, short nose, high cheeks, and feet which are not longer than a man's finger. In the Labrador Islands no woman is beautiful who has not black teeth and white hair. In Greenland and some other northern countries, the women paint their faces blue, and some yellow. Some nations squeeze the heads of children between boards to make them *square*, while others prefer the shape of a *sugar-loaf* as the highest type of beauty for that important top-piece to the "human form divine." So that there is nothing truer than the old proverb, that "there is no accounting for tastes." This difference of opinion with respect to beauty in various countries is, however, principally confined to *color* and *form*, and may, undoubtedly, be traced to national habits and customs. Nor is it fair, perhaps, to oppose the tastes of uncivilized people to the opinions of civilized nations. But then it must not be overlooked that the standard of beauty in civilized countries is by no means agreed upon. Neither the *buona roba* of the Italians, nor the *linda* of the Spaniards, nor the *embonpoint* of the French, can fully reach the mystical standard of *beauty* to the eye of American taste. And if I were to say that it consists of an indescribable combination of all these, still you would go beyond even that, before you would be content with the definition. Perhaps the best definition of beauty ever given, was by a French poet, who called it a certain *je ne sais quoi*, or, *I don't know what!*

The following classical synopsis of female beauty, which has been attributed to Félibien, is the best I remember to have seen:

"The head should be well rounded and look rather inclining to small than large.

"The forehead white, smooth, and open (not with the hair growing down too deep upon it), neither flat nor prominent, but, like the head, well rounded, and rather small in proportion than large.

"The hair either black, bright brown, or auburn, not thin, but full and waving, and if it falls in moderate curls, the better—the black is particularly useful in setting off the whiteness of the neck and skin.

"The eyes black, chestnut, or blue; clear, bright, and lively, and rather large in proportion than small.

"The eyebrows well divided, full, semicircular, and broader in the middle than at the ends, of a neat turn, but not formal.

"The cheeks should not be wide, should have a degree of plumpness, with the red and white finely blended together, and should look firm and soft.

"The ear should be rather small, well folded, and have an agreeable tinge of red.

"The nose should be placed so as to divide the face into equal parts; should be of a moderate size, straight, and well squared, though sometimes a little rising in the middle, which is just perceivable, may give a very graceful look to it.

"The mouth should be small, and the lips not of equal thickness; they should be well turned, small, rather than gross, soft even to the eye, and with a living red in them; a truly pretty mouth is like a rosebud that is beginning to blow. The teeth should be middle-sized, white, well ranged and even.

"The chin of a moderate size, white, soft, and agreeably rounded.

"The neck should be white, straight, and of a soft, easy, flexible make; rather long than short, less above, and increasing gently towards the shoulders; the whiteness and delicacy of its skin should be continued, or rather go on improving to the bosom; the skin in general should be white, properly tinged with red, and a look of thriving health in it.

"The shoulders should be white, gently spread, and

with a much softer appearance of strength than in those of men.

"The arm should be white, round, firm and soft, and more particularly so from the elbow to the hand.

"The hand should unite insensibly with the arm; it should be long and delicate, and even the joints and nervous parts of it should be without either any hardness or dryness.

"The fingers should be fine, long, round and soft; small and lessening to the tips, and the nails rather long, round at the ends, and pellucid.

"The bosom should be white and charming, neither too large nor too small; the breasts equal in roundness and firmness, rising gently, and very distinctly separated.

"The sides should be rather long and the hips wider than the shoulders, and go down rounding and lessening gradually to the knee.

"The knee should be even and well rounded.

"The legs straight but varied by proper rounding of the more fleshy parts of them, and finely turned, white, and small at the ankle."

It is very fortunate, however, for the human race that all men do not have exactly a correct taste in the matter of female beauty, for if they had, a fatal degree of strife would be likely to ensue as to who should possess the few types of perfect beauty. The old man who rejoiced that all did not see alike, as, if they did, all would be after his wife, was not far out of the way.

CHAPTER II

A HANDSOME FORM

*M*any women who can lay no claims to a beautiful face have carried captive the hearts of plenty of men by the beauty of their form. Indeed it may be questioned if a perfect form does not possess a power of captivation beyond any charms that the most beautiful face possesses. You will often hear men say of such and such a girl, "to be sure she has not a beautiful face, but then she has a most exquisite form;" and this they speak with such a peculiar earnestness that it is quite evident they mean what they say.

Those gloomy and ascetic beings who contemn the human body as only a cumbersome lump of clay, as a piece of corruption, and as the charnel-house of the soul, insult their maker, by despising the most ingenious and beautiful piece of mechanism of his physical creation. God has displayed so much care and love upon our bodies that He not only created them for usefulness, but he adorned them with loveliness. If it was not beneath our maker's glory to frame them in beauty, it certainly cannot be beneath us to respect and preserve the charms which we have received from his loving hand. To slight these gifts is to despise the giver. He that has made the temple of our souls beautiful, certainly would not have us neglect the means of preserving that beauty. Every woman owes it not only to herself, but to society, to be as beautiful and charming as she possibly can. The popular cant about the *beauty of the mind* as something which is inconsistent with, and in opposition to the *beauty of the body*, is a superstition which cannot be for a moment entertained by any sound and rational mind. To despise the *temple* is to insult its *occupant*. The divine intelligence which has planted the roses of beauty in the human cheeks, and lighted its fires in the eyes, has also entrusted us with a mission to multiply and increase these charms, as well as to develop and educate our intellects.

Let every woman feel, then, that so far from doing wrong, she is in the pleasant ways of duty when she is studying how to develop and preserve the natural beauty of her body.

> "There's nothing ill can dwell in such a temple:
> If the ill spirit have so fair a house,
> Good things will strive to dwell with it."
>
> Shakespeare.

CHAPTER III

HOW TO OBTAIN

A HANDSOME FORM

*T*he foundation for a beautiful form must undoubtedly be laid in infancy. That is, nothing should be done at that tender age to obstruct the natural swell and growth of all the parts. "As the twig is bent, the tree's inclined," is quite as true of the *body* as of the *mind*. Common sense teaches us that the young fibres ought to be left, unencumbered by obstacles of art, to shoot harmoniously into the shape that nature drew. But this is a business for mothers to attend to.

It is important, however, that the girl should understand, as soon as she comes to the years of discretion, or as soon as she is old enough to realize the importance of beauty to a woman, that she has, to a certain extent, the management of her own form within her power. The first thing to be thought of is *health*, for there can be no development of beauty in sickly fibres. Plenty of exercise, in the open air, is the great recipe. Exercise, not philosophically and with religious gravity undertaken, but the wild romping activities of a spirited girl who runs up and down as though her veins were full of wine. Everything should be done to give joy and vivacity to the spirits at this age, for nothing so much aids in giving vigor and elasticity to the form as these. A crushed, or sad, or moping spirit, allowed at this tender age, when the shape is forming, is a fatal cause of a flabby and moping body. A bent and stooping form is quite sure to come of a bent and stooping spirit. If you would have the shape "sway gracefully on the firmly poised waist"—if you would see the chest rise and swell in noble and healthy expansion, send out the girl to constant and vigorous exercise in the open air.

And, what is good for the *girl* is good for the *woman*, too. The same attention to the laws of *health*, and the same pursuit of out-door exercise will help a lady to develop a handsome form until she is twenty or twenty-five years old. "Many a rich lady would give all her fortune to possess the expanded chest and rounded arm of her kitchen girl. Well, she might have had both, by the same amount of exercise and spare living." And she can do much to acquire them even yet.

There have been many instances of sedentary men, of shrunk and sickly forms, with deficient muscle and scraggy arms, who by a change of business to a vigorous out-door exercise acquired fine robust forms, with arms as powerful and muscular as Hercules himself. I knew a young lady, who, at twenty-two years of age, in a great degree overcame the deformity of bad arms. In every other respect she was a most bewitching beauty. But her arms were distressingly thin and scraggy; and she determined at whatever pains, to remedy the evil. She began by a strict adherence to such a strong nutritious diet as was most favorable to the creation of muscle. She walked every day several hours in the open air, and never neglected the constant daily use of the dumb-bells. Thus she kept on, exercising and drilling herself, for two years, when a visible improvement showed itself, in the straightened and expanded chest; and in the fine hard swell of muscle upon the once deformed arms. She had fought, and she had conquered. Her perseverance was abundantly rewarded. Let the lady, who is ambitious for such charms, be assured that, if she has them not, they can be obtained on no lighter conditions.

CHAPTER IV

HOW TO ACQUIRE A BRIGHT

AND SMOOTH SKIN

*T*he most perfect form will avail a woman little, unless it possess also that *brightness* which is the finishing touch and final polish of a beautiful lady. What avails a plump and well-rounded neck or shoulder if it is dim and dingy withal? What charm can be found in the finest modelled arm if its skin is coarse and rusty? A *grater*, even though moulded in the shape of the most charming female arm, would possess small attractions to a man of taste and refinement.

I have to tell you, ladies—and the same must be said to the gentlemen, too—that the great secret of acquiring a bright and beautiful skin lies in three simple things, as I have said in my lecture on Beautiful Women—temperance, exercise, and cleanliness. A young lady, were she as fair as Hebe, as charming as Venus herself, would soon destroy it all by too high living and late hours. "Take the ordinary fare of a fashionable woman, and you have a style of living which is sufficient to destroy the greatest beauty. It is not the *quantity* so much as the *quality* of the dishes that produces the mischief. Take, for instance, only strong coffee and hot bread and butter, and you have a diet which is most destructive to beauty. The heated grease, long indulged in, is sure to derange the stomach, and, by creating or increasing bilious disorders, gradually overspreads the fair skin with a wan or yellow hue. After this meal comes the long fast from nine in the morning till five or six in the afternoon, when dinner is served, and the half-famished beauty sits down to sate a keen appetite with peppered soups, fish, roast, boiled, broiled, and fried meat; game, tarts, sweet-meats, ices, fruits, etc., etc., etc. How must the constitution suffer in trying to digest this *mélange!* How does the heated complexion bear witness to the combustion within! Let the fashionable lady keep up this habit, and add the other one of late hours, and her own looking-glass will tell her that 'we all do fade as the leaf.' The firm texture of the rounded form gives way to a flabby softness, or yields to a scraggy leanness, or shapeless fate. The once fair skin assumes a pallid rigidity or bloated redness, which the deluded victim would still regard as the roses of health and beauty. And when she at last becomes aware of her condition, to repair the ravages she flies to paddings, to give shape where there is none; to stays, to compress into form the swelling chaos of flesh; and to paints, to rectify the dingy complexion. But vain are all these attempts. No; if dissipation, late hours, and immoderation have once wrecked the fair vessel of female charms, it is not in the power of Esculapius himself to right the shattered bark, and make it ride the sea in gallant trim again." *

Cleanliness is a subject of indispensable consideration in the pursuit of a beautiful skin. The frequent use of the tepid bath is the best cosmetic I can recommend to my readers in this connection. By such ablutions, the acci-

* *My Lecture on Beautiful Women.*

dental corporeal impurities are thrown off, cutaneous obstructions removed; and while the surface of the body is preserved in its original brightness, many threatening disorders are prevented. It is by this means that the women of the East render their skins as soft and fair as those of the tenderest babes. I wish to impress upon every beautiful woman, and especially upon the one who leads a city life, that she cannot long preserve the brightness of her charms without a daily resort to this purifying agent. She should make the bath as indispensable an article in her house as her looking-glass.

CHAPTER V

ARTIFICIAL MEANS

esides the rational and natural means of developing and preserving the beauty of the skin, there are many artificial devices by which a lady may keep up and show off her attractions to great advantage, and for a long period.

As long ago as 1809, an odd and half-crazy old duke in London, used to take a sweat in a hot-milk bath, which was found to impart a remarkable whiteness and smoothness to his skin, and the ladies very naturally caught the idea of using the milk-bath as a means of beautifying their complexion. In another place I have mentioned some ludicrous scenes which followed the habit of milk-bathing in Paris.

But a far more rational, less expensive, and more scientific bath for cleaning and beautifying the skin is that of tepid water and bran, which is really a remarkably fine softener and purifyer of the surface of the body.

The ladies of ancient Greece and Rome, who were said to be remarkable for the brightness and transparency of their skins, used to rub themselves with a sponge, dampened with cold water, and follow this process by rubbing hard with a dry napkin. Rightly managed, the human skin is susceptible of a high polish. *Friction* is never to be neglected by those who would *shine* in the courts of beauty.

The following wash was in great use among the beauties of the Spanish Court, and gives a polished whiteness to the neck and arms.

Infuse wheat-bran, well sifted, for four hours in white wine vinegar; add to it five yolks of eggs and two grains of ambergris, and distill the whole. It should be carefully corked for twelve or fifteen days, when it will be fit for use.

A lady may apply it every time she makes her toilet, and it will be sure to add a fine polish and lustre to her skin.

The following wash is a great favorite with the ladies on the continent of Europe, and cannot be used without the happiest effects, while it is a delightful and refreshing perfume:

Distill two handfuls of jessamine flowers in a quart of rose-water and a quart of orange-water. Strain through porous paper, and add a scruple of musk and a scruple of ambergris.

There cannot be a more agreeable wash for the skin.

CHAPTER VI

BEAUTY OF ELASTICITY

*T*he most perfect form, and the most brilliant skin will avail a woman little, unless she possess, also, that physical *agility*, or elasticity, which is the *soul* of a beautiful form in woman. A half-alive and sluggish body, however perfectly formed, is, to say the most, but half beautiful. When you behold a woman who is like a wood-nymph, with a form elastic in all its parts, and a foot as light as that of the goddess, whose flying step "scarcely brushed the unbending corn," whose conscious limbs and agile grace moved in harmony with the light of her sparkling eyes, you may be sure that she carries all hearts before her. There are women whose exquisite forms seem as flexible, wavy and undulating as the graceful lilies of the field. The stiff and prim city belle, encased in hoops and buckram, may well envy that agile, bouncing country romp, who, with nature's roses in her cheeks, skips it like a fawn, and sends out a laugh as natural and merry as the notes of song-birds in June. And she may be sure that her husband or lover never looks upon such a specimen of nature's own beauty, but that he quietly wishes in his heart that his wife, or sweetheart, were like her. Let the city belle learn a lesson from this. She can have the same charms on the same conditions that the country lass has obtained them. But, by high living, late hours, and all the other dissipations of fashionable city life—*never!* That country lass goes to bed with the robin and is up with the lark. Her life is after nature's fashion, and she is rewarded with nature's most sprightly gifts. Whereas this city belle goes to bed at indefinite midnight hours, and crawls languidly out at mid-day, with a jaded body and a feverish mind, to mope through the tedious rounds of daily dullness, until night again rallies her faint and exhausted spirits. Her life is by gaslight.

Most that I have said in the chapter on the means of obtaining a bright and handsome form, applies equally to the subject of this chapter. But, there are some artificial tricks which I have known beautiful ladies to resort to for the purpose of giving elasticity and sprightliness to the animal frame. The ladies of France and Italy, especially those who are professionally, or as amateurs, engaged in exercises which require great activity of the limbs, as dancing, or playing on instruments, sometimes rub themselves, on retiring to bed, with the following preparation:

> Fat of the stag, or deer . . . 8 oz.
> Florence oil (or olive oil) . . 6 oz.
> Virgin wax . . . . 3 oz.
> Musk . . . . 1 grain.
> White brandy . . . . ½ pint.
> Rose-water . . . . 4 oz.

Put the fat, oil, and wax into a well-glazed earthen vessel, and let them simmer over a slow fire until they are assimilated; then pour in the other ingredients, and let the whole gradually cool, when it will be fit for use. There is no doubt but that this mixture, frequently and thoroughly rubbed upon the body on going to bed, will impart a remarkable degree of elasticity to the muscles. In the morning, after this preparation has been used, the body should be thoroughly wiped with a sponge, dampened with cold water.

CHAPTER VII

A BEAUTIFUL FACE

*I*f it be true "that the face is the index of the mind," the recipe for a beautiful face must be something that reaches the soul. What can be done for a human face that has a sluggish, sullen, arrogant, angry mind looking out of every feature? An habitually ill-natured, discontented mind ploughs the face with inevitable marks of its own vice. However well shaped, or however bright its complexion, no such face can ever become really beautiful. If a woman's soul is without cultivation, without taste, without refinement, without the sweetness of a happy mind, not all the mysteries of art can ever make her face beautiful. And, on the other hand, it is impossible to dim the brightness of an elegant and polished intellect. The radiance of a charming mind strikes through all deformity of features, and still asserts its sway over the world of the affections. It has been my privilege to see the most celebrated beauties that shine in all the gilded courts of fashion throughout the world from St. James's to St. Petersburgh, from Paris to Hindostan, and yet I have found no art which can atone for an unpolished mind, and an unlovely heart. That chastened and delightful activity of soul, that spiritual energy which gives animation, grace, and living light to the animal frame, is, after all, the real source of beauty in a woman. It is *that* which gives eloquence to the language of her eyes, which sends the sweetest vermilion mantling to the cheek, and lights up the whole *personnel* as if her very body thought. That, ladies, is the ensign of beauty, and the herald of charms, which are sure to fill the beholder with answering emotion, and irrepressible delight. I never see a creature of such lively and lovely animation, but I fall in love with her myself, and only wish that I were a man, that I might marry her.*

I cannot resist the temptation to close this chapter with a beautiful quotation from an old Greek poet, which proves that common sense on this subject of beauty is not by any means of recent date in the world.

> *"Why tinge the cheek of youth? the snowy neck,*
> *Why load with jewels? why anoint the hair?*
> *Oh, lady, scorn these arts; but richly deck*
> *Thy soul with virtues: thus for love prepare.*
> *Lo, with what vermil tints the apple blooms!*
> *Say, doth the rose the painter's hand require?*
> *Away, then, with cosmetics and perfumes!*
> *The charms of nature most excite desire."*

* *Lecture on Beautiful Women.*

CHAPTER VIII

HOW TO OBTAIN

A BEAUTIFUL COMPLEXION

hough it is true that a beautiful mind is the first thing requisite for a beautiful face, yet how much more charming will the whole become through the aid of a fine complexion? It is not easy to overrate the importance of *complexion*. The features of a Juno with a dull skin would never fascinate. The forehead, the nose, the lips, may all be faultless in size and shape; but still, they can hardly look beautiful without the aid of a bright complexion. Even the finest eyes lose more than half their power, if they are surrounded by an inexpressive complexion. It is in the *coloring* or *complexion* that the artist shows his great skill in giving expression to the face. Overlooking entirely the matter of *vanity*, it is a woman's *duty* to use all the means in her power to beautify and preserve her complexion. It is fitting that the "index of the soul" should be kept as clean and bright and beautiful as possible.

All that I have said in chapters IV. and V., apply also to the subject of the present chapter. A stomach frequently crowded with greasy food, or with artificial stimulants of any kind, will in a short time spoil the brightest complexion. All *excesses* tend to do the same thing. Frequent ablution with pure cold water, followed by gentle and very frequent rubbing with a dry napkin, is one of the best cosmetics ever employed.

It is amusing to reflect upon the tricks which vain beauties will resort to in order to obtain this paramount aid to female charms. Nor is it any wonder that woman should exhaust all her resources in this pursuit, for her face is such a public thing, that there is no hiding the least deformity in it. She can, to some extent, hide an ugly neck, or shoulder, or hand, or foot—but there is no hiding-place for an ugly face.

I knew many fashionable ladies in Paris who used to bind their faces, every night on going to bed, with thin slices of raw beef, which is said to keep the skin from wrinkles, while it gives a youthful freshness and brilliancy to the complexion. I have no doubt of its efficacy. The celebrated Madam Vestris used to sleep every night with her face plastered up with a kind of paste to ward off the threatening wrinkles, and keep her charming complexion from fading. I will give the recipe for making the Vestris' Paste for the benefit of any of my readers whose looking-glass warns them that the dimness and wrinkles of age are extinguishing the roses of youth:

The whites of four eggs boiled in rose-water, half an ounce of alum, half an ounce of oil of sweet almonds; beat the whole together till it assumes the consistence of a paste.

The above, spread upon a silk or muslin mask, and worn at night, will not only keep back the wrinkles and preserve the complexion fair, but it is a great remedy where the skin becomes too loosely attached to the muscles, as it gives firmness to the parts. When I was last in

Paris (1857) I was shown a recent invention of ready-made masks for the face, composed of fine thick white silk, lined, or plastered, with some kind of fard, or paste, which is designed to beautify and preserve the complexion. I do not know the component parts of this preparation; but I doubt if it is any better than the recipe which was given to me by Madam Vestris, and which I have given above. This trick is so entirely French that there is little danger of its getting into *general* practice in this country. In Bohemia I have seen the ladies flock to arsenic springs and drink the waters, which gave their skins a transparent whiteness; but there is a terrible penalty attached to this folly; for when once they habituate themselves to the practice, they are obliged to keep it up the rest of their days, or death would speedily follow. The beauties of the court of George I. were in the habit of taking minute doses of quicksilver to obtain a white and fair complexion; and I have read in Pepys's Diary of some ridiculous scenes which occurred at dancing parties from this practice. Young girls of the present day sometimes eat such things as chalk, slate, and tea-grounds to give themselves a white complexion. I have no doubt that this is a good way to get a *pale* complexion; for it destroys the health, and surely drives out of the face the natural roses of beauty, and, instead of a bright complexion, produces a wan and sickly one. Every young girl ought early to be impressed that whatever destroys health spoils her beauty.

The most remarkable wash for the face which I have ever known, and which is said to have been known to the beauties of the court of Charles II., is made of a simple tincture of *benzoin* precipitated by water. All you have to do in preparing it is to *take a small piece of the gum benzoin and boil it in spirits of wine till it becomes a rich tincture. Fifteen drops of this, poured into a glass of water, will produce a mixture which will look like milk, and emits a most agreeable perfume.*

This delightful wash seems to have the effect of calling the purple stream of the blood to the external fibres of the face, and gives the cheeks a beautiful rosy color. If left on the face to dry, it will render the skin clear and brilliant. It is also an excellent remedy for spots, freckles, pimples, and eruptions, if they have not been of long standing.

CHAPTER IX

HABITS WHICH DESTROY

THE COMPLEXION

*T*here are many disorders of the skin which are induced by culpable ignorance, and which owe their origin entirely to circumstances connected with *fashion* or *habit*. The frequent and sudden changes in this country from heat to cold, by abruptly exciting or repressing the secretions of the skin, roughen its texture, injure its hue, and often deform it with unseemly eruptions. And many of the fashions of dressing the head, are still more inimical to the complexion, than the climate. The habit the ladies have of going into the open air without a bonnet, and often without a veil, is a ruinous one for the skin. Indeed, the fashion of the ladies' bonnets, which only cover a few inches of the back of the head, is a great tax upon the beauty of the complexion. In this climate, especially, the head and face need protection from the atmosphere. Not only a woman's *beauty*, but her *health* requires that she should never step into the open air, particularly in autumnal evenings, without a sufficient covering to her head. And, if she regards the beauty of her complexion, she must never go out into the hot sun without her veil.

The custom, common among ladies, of drying the perspiration from their faces by powdering, or of cooling them when they are hot, from exposure to the sun or dancing, by washing with cold water, is most destructive to the complexion, and not unfrequently spreads a humor over the face which renders it hideous forever. A little common sense ought to teach a woman that, when she is overheated, she ought to allow herself to cool gradually; and, by all means, to avoid going into the air, or allowing a draught through an open door, or window, to blow upon her while she is thus heated. If she will not attend to these rules, she will be fortunate, saying nothing about her beauty, if her *life* does not pay the penalty of her thoughtlessness.

Ladies ought also to know that excessive heat is as bad as excessive cold for the complexion, and often causes distempers of the skin, which are difficult of cure. Look at the rough and dingy face of the desert-wandering gipsy, and you behold the effects of exposure to alternate heats and colds.

To remedy the rigidity of the muscles of the face, and to cure any roughness which may be induced by daily exposure, the following wash may be applied with almost certain relief:

Mix two parts of white brandy with one part of rose-water, and wash the face with it night and morning.

The brandy keeps up a gentle action of the skin, which is so essential to its healthy appearance, also thoroughly cleanses the surface, while the rose-water counteracts the drying nature of the brandy, and leaves the skin in a natural, soft, and flexible state.

At a trifling expense, a lady may provide herself with a delightful wash for the face, which is a thousand times

better than the expensive *lotions* which she purchases at
the apothecaries. Besides, she has the advantage of know-
ing what she is using, which is far from being the case
where she buys the prepared patent lotions. These preparations are generally put up by ignorant quacks and
pretenders; and I have known the most loathsome,
beauty-destroying, indolent ulcers to be produced by the
use of them.

The following is a recipe for making another wash for
the face, which is a favorite with the ladies of France.

*Take equal parts of the seeds of the melon, pumpkin,
gourd and cucumber, pounded till they are reduced to
powder; add to it sufficient fresh cream to dilute the
flour, and then add milk enough to reduce the whole to a
thin paste. Add a grain of musk, and a few drops of the
oil of lemon. Anoint the face with this, leave it on twenty
or thirty minutes, or overnight if convenient, and wash
off with warm water. It gives a remarkable purity and
brightness to the complexion.*

A fashionable beauty at St. Petersburgh gave me the
following recipe for a wash, which imparts a remarkable
lustre to the face, and is the greatest favorite of a Russian
lady's toilet.

*Infuse a handful of well sifted wheat-bran for four
hours in white wine vinegar; add to it five yolks of eggs
and two grains of musk, and distill the whole. Bottle it,
keep carefully corked, fifteen days, when it will be fit for
use. Apply it overnight, and wash in the morning with
tepid water.*

Pimpernel Water is a sovereign wash with the ladies
all over the continent of Europe, for whitening the complexion. All they do to prepare it is simply to steep that

wholesome plant in pure rain water. It is such a favorite that it is regarded as almost indispensable to a lady's toilet, who is particularly attentive to the brightness of her complexion.

CHAPTER X

PAINTS AND POWDERS

*I*f Satan has ever had any direct agency in inducing woman to spoil or deform her own beauty, it must have been in tempting her to use *paints* and *enamelling*. Nothing so effectually writes *memento mori!* on the cheek of beauty as this ridiculous and culpable practice. Ladies ought to know that it is a sure spoiler of the skin, and good taste ought to teach them that it is a frightful distorter and deformer of the natural beauty of the "human face divine." The greatest charm of beauty is in the *expression* of a lovely face; in those divine flashes of joy, and good-nature, and love, which beam in the human countenance. But what expression can there be in "a face bedaubed with white paint and enamelled? No flush of pleasure, no thrill of hope, no light of love can shine through the encrusted mould." Her face is as expressionless as that of a painted mummy. And let no woman imagine that the men do not readily detect this poisonous mask upon the skin. Many a time have I seen a gentleman shrink from saluting a brilliant lady, as though it was a death's head he were compelled to kiss. The secret was, that her face and lips were bedaubed with paints. All white paints are not only destructive to the skin, but they are ruinous to the health. I have known paralytic affections and premature death to be traced to their use. But alas! I am afraid that there never was a time when many of the gay and fashionable of my sex, did not make themselves both contemptible and ridiculous by this disgusting trick. The ancient ladies seem to have outdone even modern belles in this painting business. The terrible old Juvenal draws the following picture of one of the flirts of his day.

> *"But tell me yet; this thing, thus daubed and oiled,*
> *Poulticed, plastered, baked by turns, and boiled,*
> *Thus with pomatums, ointments, lacquered o'er,*
> *Is it a face, Usidius, or a sore?"*

But it is proper to remark, that what has been said against white paint and enamels does not apply with equal force to the use of *rouge*. Rouging still leaves the neck and arms, and more than three-quarters of the face to their natural complexion, and the language of the heart, expressed by the general complexion, is not obstructed. A little vegetable *rouge* tinging the cheek of a beautiful woman, who, from ill health or an anxious mind, loses her roses, may be excusable; and so transparent is the texture of such *rouge* (if unadulterated with lead) than when the blood does mount to the face, it speaks through the slight covering, and enhances the fading bloom. But even this allowable artificial aid must be used with the most delicate taste, and discretion. The tint on the cheek should always be fainter than what nature's pallet would have painted. A violently rouged woman is a disgusting sight. The excessive red on the face gives a coarseness to every feature, and a general fierceness to the countenance, which transforms the elegant lady of fashion into a vulgar harridan. But, in no case, can even *rouge* be used by ladies who have passed the age of life when roses are natural to the cheek. A *rouged* old woman is a horrible sight—a distortion of nature's harmony!

Excessive use of *powder* is also a vulgar trick. None but the very finest powder should ever be used, and the lady should be especially careful that sufficient is not left upon the face to be noticeable to the eye of a gentleman. She must be very particular that particles of it are not left visible about the base of the nose, and in the hollow of the chin. Ladies sometimes catch up their powder, and rub it on in a hurry, without even stopping to look in the glass, and go into company with their faces looking as though they just came out of a meal-bag. It is a ridiculous sight, and ladies may be sure it is disgusting to gentlemen.

CHAPTER XI

A BEAUTIFUL BOSOM

I am aware that this is a subject which must be handled with great delicacy; but my book would be incomplete without some notice of this "greatest claim of lovely woman." And, besides, it is undoubtedly true that a proper discussion of this subject will seem *peculiar* only to the most vulgar minded of both sexes. If it be true, as the old poet sang, that

"Heaven rests on those two heaving hills of snow,"

why should not a woman be suitably instructed in the right management of such extraordinary charms?

The first thing to be impressed upon the mind of a lady is, that very low-necked dresses are in exceeding bad taste, and are quite sure to leave upon the mind of a gentleman an equivocal idea, to say the least. A word to the wise on this subject is sufficient. If a young lady has no father, or brother, or husband to direct her taste in this matter, she will do well to sit down and commit the above statement to memory. It is a charm which a woman, who understands herself, will leave not to the public eye of man, but to his imagination. She knows that *modesty*

is the divine spell that binds the heart of man to her forever. But my observation has taught me that few women
are well informed as to the physical management of this
part of their bodies. The bosom, which nature has formed
with exquisite symmetry in itself, and admirable adaptation to the parts of the figure to which it is united, is often
transformed into a shape, and transplanted to a place,
which deprive it of its original beauty and harmony with
the rest of the person. This deforming metamorphosis is
effected by means of stiff stays, or corsets, which force the
part out of its natural position, and destroy the natural
tension and firmness in which so much of its beauty consists. A young lady should be instructed that she is not to
allow even her own hand to press it too roughly. But,
above all things, to avoid, especially when young, the constant pressure of such hard substances as whalebone and
steel; for, besides the destruction to beauty, they are
liable to produce all the terrible consequences of abscesses
and cancers. Even the padding which ladies use to give a
full appearance, where there is a deficient bosom, is sure,
in a little time, to entirely destroy all the natural beauty
of the parts. As soon as it becomes apparent that the
bosom lacks the rounded fullness due to the rest of her
form, instead of trying to repair the deficiency with artificial padding, it should be clothed as loosely as possible,
so as to avoid the least artificial pressure. Not only its
growth is stopped, but its complexion is spoiled by these
tricks. Let the growth of this beautiful part be left as
unconfined as the young cedar, or as the lily of the field.
And for that reason the bodice should be flexible to the
motion of the body and the undulations of the shape. The
artificial india-rubber bosoms are not only ridiculous

contrivances, but they are absolutely ruinous to the beauty of the part.

The following preparation, very softly rubbed upon the bosom for five or ten minutes, two or three times a day has been used with success to promote its growth.

Tincture of myrrh	½ oz.
Pimpernel water	4 oz.
Elder-flower water	4 oz.
Musk	1 gr.
Rectified spirits of wine	6 oz.

I have known ladies to take a preparation of iodine internally to remedy a too large development of the bosom. But this must be a dangerous experiment for the general health. The following external application has been recommended for this purpose.

Strong essence of mint	1 oz.
Iodine of zinc	2 gr.
Aromatic vinegar	2 gr.
Essence of cedrat	10 drops.

If, from sickness, or any other cause, the bosom has lost its beauty by becoming soft, the following wash, applied as gently as possible morning and night, will have a most beneficial effect.

Alum water	½ oz.
Strong camomile water	1 oz.
White brandy	2 oz.

If the whole body is not afflicted with a general decay and flabbiness, the use of this wash for a month or two will be quite sure to produce the happiest effects.

CHAPTER XII

BEAUTIFUL EYES

*T*he eyes have been called the "windows of the soul," and all that I have said in another part of this book of the influence of the passions on the beauty or deformity of the face, applies with peculiar force in this place. Nowhere will ill-nature and bad passions show themselves so glancingly as in the eyes. Whenever we would find out what the soul is, we look straightway into its "windows." If they close upon us, or turn away, we are forced to conclude that all is not right within. On the other hand, where we see frank, happy, laughing eyes, we naturally believe that amiability, sincerity, and truth are in the heart. It is not so much the *color* or the *size* of the eyes, as it is their *expression* that makes them beautiful.

There is no more wretched deformity to a woman than a certain unnatural, and studied *languishing* of the eyes, which vain and silly women sometimes effect. I have read that when Sir Peter Lely painted a celebrated belle, who had the sweet peculiarity of a long and languishing eye, no fashionable lady for a long time appeared in public who did not affect the soft sleepiness and tender slow-moving look of Sir Peter's picture. The result, of course, was that queer *leers* and *squints* everywhere met a gentleman's gaze in the distorted faces of the fair. There is no one of the beautiful organs of woman that needs to be left so entirely to the unconstrained *art of nature* as the eye. Let woman believe that all the tricks played with the eyes, are absurd and ruinous to beauty. It once happened in Turkey that the monarch expressed his great admiration for "large and dark-lashed eyes." From that hour, all the fair slaves on whom nature had not bestowed "the wild stag-eye in sable ringlets rolling," set to work to supply the deficiency with circles of antimony. Thousands of beautiful women must have frightfully distorted themselves. There is, almost invariably, a lovely harmony between the color of the eyes and its fringes and the complexion of a woman, which cannot be broken up by art without an insult to nature. The fair complexion is generally accompanied with blue eyes, light hair, and light eye-brows and eye-lashes. The delicacy of one feature is preserved, in effect and beauty, by the corresponding softness of the other. But take this fair creature, and draw a black line over her softly tinctured eyes, stain their beamy fringes with a sombre hue, and how frightfully have you mutilated nature! On the other hand, a brunette with light eye-brows, would be a caricature of a beautiful woman. If a woman has the misfortune from disease, or otherwise, to have deficient eye-brows, she may delicately supply the want, as far as she can, with artificial pencilling; but, in doing this, she must scrupulously follow nature and make the color of her pencilling to correspond with her complexion. The Eastern women, many of whom have large dark eyes, have great skill in pencilling the eye so as to add to its natural power; but I have witnessed ridiculous failures in such tricks, even there. The Turkish and Circassian women use *henna* for pencilling the eyes. Among the Arabs of the desert, the women blacken the edge of their eye-lids with a black powder, and draw a line round the eye with it, to make the organ appear large. Large black eyes are the standard of beauty among nearly all Eastern women.

The Spanish ladies have a custom of squeezing orange juice into their eyes to make them brilliant. The operation is a little painful for a moment, but there is no doubt that it does cleanse the eye, and impart to it, temporarily, a remarkable brightness. But the best recipe for bright eyes is to keep good hours. Just enough regular and natural sleep is the great enkindler of "woman's most charming light."

And, before I close this chapter, let me warn ladies against the use of white veils. Scarcely anything can strain and jade and injure the eye more than this practice. There is reason to believe that the sight sometimes becomes permanently injured by them.

It is within the power of almost every lady to have long and strong eye-lashes by simply clipping, with scissors, the points of the hair once in five or six weeks.

*T*he beauty of the mouth and lips has been a rapturous theme for lovers and poets, ever since the world began. Old Hafiz, the great poet of Persia, sang perpetually of

> *"Lips that outblush the ruby's red,*
> *With luscious dews of sweetness fed."*

Even Milton's stern lyre was tuned to sweetest song about

> *"The vermil-tinctured lip."*

And Petrarch seems to have found no charm in the divine Laura greater than her "beautiful and angelical mouth." *"La bella bocca angelica!"* he exclaims. And so Dante found inexpressible delight in the charming mouth of Beatrice, especially when it said *"yes."* "Thus," says he, "it is my remembrance of that mouth of hers which spurs me on ever, since there is nothing which I would not give to hear her say, with a perfect good will, a *yes*." Yes, it is the *sentiment* or *emotion* that lingers about the mouth that constitutes much of its beauty. A mouth perpetually contracted as though it were about to say *no*, or curled up with passions of sarcasm and ill-nature, cannot be beautiful, even though its lips were chiselled like Diana's, and stained with the red of the ripest cherries. The mouth, indeed, is scarcely less expressive than the eyes, and therefore woman must not forget that its chief beauty consists in the *expression*. If a lady is anxious to have her mouth look particularly charming for some particular occasion, she will do well to fill her thoughts with some very delightful subject. And let her not forget that the muscles of the mouth and face are, like the rest of human nature, "creatures of habit;" and long use in the language of amiability and happiness, gives that expressive organ its greatest charm. An old Persian poet sings to his beloved:

> *"The language anger prompts I bear;*
> *If kind thy speech, I bless my fair;*
> *But, is it fit that words of gall*
> *From lovely lips, like thine, should fall?"*

Let every woman at once understand that paint can do nothing for the mouth and lips. The advantage gained by the artificial red is a thousand times more than lost by the sure destruction of that delicate charm associated with the idea of "nature's dewy lip." There can be no *dew* on a painted lip. And there is no man who does not shrink back with disgust from the idea of kissing a pair of painted lips. Nor let any woman deceive herself with the idea that the men do not instantly detect paint on her lips.

Ruby lips are generally the result and the ensign of

perfect health. But, still, those who are entirely well do not always enjoy the possession of cherry lips. Where this is the case, the tincture of benzoin, as described in Chapter VIII and which has none of the properties of paint, may be used with beneficial effects. I need not remind the ladies that clean white teeth are indispensable to a beautiful mouth. The lady who neglects to brush her teeth with pure cold water after every meal, not only loses the benefit of the natural whiteness of her teeth but she renders herself liable to have the disgusting evil of an impure breath. The best tooth-powder I know of is made as follows:

> Prepared chalk . . 6 oz.
> Cassia powder . . . ½ oz.
> Orris-root . . . . . 1 oz.

These should be thoroughly mixed and used once a day with a firm brush.

A simple mixture of charcoal and cream of tartar is an excellent tooth-powder.

To be sure of a sweet and clean-looking mouth, a lady should take her looking-glass after each meal and with a fine tooth-pick gently remove the particles of food, or any matter, which may be discovered about the roots of the teeth, or in the interstices. To ensure the great charm of a beautiful mouth requires unremitting attention to the health of the teeth and gums. To keep the gums red and firm frequent friction with the brush will be necessary.

CHAPTER XIV

A BEAUTIFUL HAND

A beautiful hand performs a great mission in the life of a belle. Indeed, the hand has a language of its own, which is often most intelligible when the tongue and every other part of the human body is compelled to be mute. When timid lovers have never dared to open their mouths to each other, their hands will get together and express all the passion that glows within. Or, often when two lovers are annoyed by the presence of a rigid mother, or guardian, they secretly squeeze each other's hands, which says, loud enough for their hearts to hear, "what a pity we are not alone!" And, when parting in the presence of the crowd, how much is said, how much promised in that gentle pressure of the hands! When a lady lets her fingers softly linger in the palm of a gentleman, what else does it say but, "you have my heart already."

But besides this secret and potent language of the hand, it is a great ornament as a thing of beauty. The great Petrarch confesses that Laura's "beautiful hand made captive his heart;" and there is no woman who is not conscious of the power she has in the possession of a charming hand.

The Spanish ladies take, if possible, more pains with

their *hands* than with their *faces*. There is no end of the tricks to which they resort to render this organ delicate and beautiful. Some of these devices are not only painful, but exceedingly ridiculous. For instance, I have known some of them to sleep every night with their hands held up to the bed-posts by pulleys, hoping by that means to render them pale and delicate. Both Spanish and French women—those at least who are very particular to make the most of these charms—are in the habit of sleeping in gloves which are lined or plastered over with a kind of pomade to improve the delicacy and complexion of their hands. This paste is generally made of the following ingredients.

Take half a pound of soft soap, a gill of salad oil, an ounce of mutton tallow, and boil them till they are thoroughly mixed. After the boiling has ceased, but before it is cold, add one gill of spirits of wine, and a grain of musk.

If any lady wishes to try this, she can buy a pair of gloves three or four sizes larger than the hand, rip them open and spread on a thin layer of the paste, and then sew the gloves up again. There is no doubt that by wearing them every night they will give smoothness and a fine complexion to the hands. Those who have the means can send to Paris and purchase them ready made. But I am not aware that they have been imported to this country. It will not surprise me, however, to learn that they *have* been, for fashionable ladies are remarkably quick at finding out the tricks which the belles elsewhere resort to for the purpose of beautifying themselves. Sleeping in simple white kid gloves will make the skin of the hand white and soft. Of course, no lady who wishes to be particular about her hands, will ever go out into the air without her gloves.

It requires almost as much labor and attention to keep the hands in order as it does to preserve the beauty of the face; taking care of the nails, alone, is an art which few women understand, for eight out of ten of even fashionable ladies always appear with their nails neither tastefully trimmed nor otherwise in good condition. The nail, properly managed, will be smooth, transparent and nearly rose-colored.

If the hands are inclined to be rough and to chap, the following wash will remedy the evil.

Lemon juice	3 oz.
White wine vinegar . .	3 oz.
White brandy	½ pint.

CHAPTER XV

A BEAUTIFUL FOOT

AND ANKLE

*I*t will be difficult to over-estimate the importance of a well-proportioned foot and ankle as a part of female beauty. There is a delightful promise in a fine foot and ankle that the rest of the limb is shaped with the same exquisite grace. And, on the other hand, a clumsy foot and ankle seems to presage a heavy and bad-shaped leg. This rule may not always be just, but there is no getting such an association out of a gentleman's mind. When was the time that the poets did not sing of the charms of a "nimble foot?" or of

> *"The fairy foot*
> *Which shines like snow, and falls on earth as mute."*

Virgil tells us that

> *"By her gentle walk, the queen of love is known,"*

and that "gentle walk" will rarely, if ever, be found connected with a heavy and an ill-shaped foot and ankle. We know it is natural for the mind to associate every other charm with that of a graceful step. Thus Milton sang—

"Grace was in all her steps, heaven in her eyes,
In every gesture dignity and love."

The pains which some nations take to ensure a small foot amounts to a torture which ought to be called by no other name than that of the *art of deforming*. In China, especially, this thing is carried to such an extent that the women's feet are entirely spoiled. In Spain, however, the art is practised with astonishing success in causing beautifully small feet. I have known ladies there, who were past twenty years of age, to sleep every night with bandages on their feet and ankles drawn as tight as they could be and not stop the circulation. There is nothing that a Spanish beauty is more proud of, than a small and beautiful foot and ankle, and nowhere do you find more of those charms than in Spain.

A great cause of thick ankles among women of the cities, who are fashionably and genteelly brought up, is a want of exercise and sitting indolently in over-heated rooms. Such habits are quite sure to produce slight swellings of the ankles, and cause a chronic flabbiness of the muscles. You might as well expect to see a rose-bush spring, bud and bloom, in a closely-pent oven, as to anticipate fine and healthy proportions from a long continuance of such habits. Let every lady be assured that there is no part of her body which will suffer more from want of proper exercise than her feet and ankles.

But woman's chief art, in making the most out of this portion of her charms, must consist in properly and tastefully dressing them. Let her start with the maxim that she had better wear a bad bonnet, than a bad shoe. Let her believe that an ill-fitting dress will not do so much towards breaking the charm of her beauty in the mind of a man, as a loose and soiled stocking.

The celebrated Madam Vestris used to have her white satin boots sewed on her feet every morning, in order that they should perfectly fit the exquisite shape of her foot. Of course, they had to be ripped off at night, and the same pair could never be worn but once. This famous beauty rejoiced in the reputation of having the handsomest foot of any woman in the world, and it was said that she made more conquests with her *feet* than with her *face*, beautiful as it was.

If a lady has not a naturally beautiful foot, her care is directed to the means of preventing attention from being called to it. For this reason, she dresses it as neatly, but as soberly as possible. Her hope is in a plain black shoe, and she especially eschews all gay colors, and all ornaments, which would be sure to attract the eye to a spot of which she cannot be proud. Indeed, bright-colored shoes are in bad taste for anybody, except on certain brilliant occasions, where fancy dresses are worn.

Above all things, every lady of taste avoids an ornamented stocking. Stockings with open-wove, ornamented insteps, denote a vulgar taste, and, instead of displaying a fine proportion, confuse the contour of a pretty foot. But, where the ankle is rather large, or square, a pretty, unobtrusive net clock, of the same color as the stocking, will be a useful device, and induce the beholder to believe in the perfect symmetry of the parts.

Though a woman is to be fully conscious of the charm of a pretty foot and ankle, yet she must not seem to be so. Nothing will draw the laugh on her so quick as a manifestly designed exhibition of these parts. It is, no doubt, a very difficult thing for a lady who has a fine foot to keep it from creeping forth into sight beneath the dress; but, let her be sure that the charm is gone the moment the beholder detects it is done designedly. If men are not modest themselves, they will never forgive a woman if she is not.

Before leaving this subject, I must not forget to speak of the importance to a lady of a genteel and sprightly *walk*. The practised eye detects the quality of a woman's mind and heart in her step. Nor is this an idle fancy, for the reason that every situation of the soul, every internal movement, has its regular progression, in the external action of the body. We may say as Seneca makes the wife of Hercules say of Lychas—

"His mind is like his walk."

An indistinct, shuffling, irregular, sluggish, and slovenly walk is a tolerably sure sign of corresponding attributes of the soul. And, on the other hand, an affected, pert, vain, and pedantic step draws upon a woman the worst impressions from the opposite gender. But there is a remarkable charm in a walk characterized by blended *dignity and vivacity*. It leaves upon the beholder a lasting impression of those attributes of mind which most surely awaken esteem and admiration.

ne of the most powerful auxiliaries of beauty is a fine, well trained voice. Indeed, one of the most fascinating women I ever knew had scarcely any other charm to recommend her. She was a young countess in Berlin, who had dull eyes, a rough skin, with dingy complexion, coarse, dull hair, and a dumpy form. But she had an exquisite voice, which charmed everybody who heard it. Ugly as she was, she was called "the syren," from the fascinating sweetness of her voice. And with an infallible instinct that she had but a single charm, she had cultivated that until she had brought it to the utmost perfection. Words fell like charmed music from her lips. And then, besides the discipline she had given her voice, she had made herself master of the art of conversation. In this respect, every woman's education is sadly neglected. Had I a daughter, the first thing I should teach her, in the way of artificial accomplishments, would be, that *to converse charmingly* is a far greater accomplishment to a lady than music and dancing. A woman who can converse well is always sure to command respect and admiration in any society. By this I, of course, don't mean a vicious abundance of words, and rapid volubility of tongue, for these are things which my sex sometimes too easily acquire. Good conversation does not mean the art of *talking*, but, the art of *talking well*. How few ladies have it! How few have ever been taught that good talking is as much an *art* as good singing? How few know that the voice can be as much improved for the art of conversation, as it can for the art of singing? It is the voice, after all, more than words, that gives the finest and clearest expression to the passions and sentiments of the soul. The most correct and elegant language loses all its beauty with a bad or ill-trained voice. The exhilaration of mirth, the profound sighs of sadness, the tenderness of love, the trembling interrupted sobbing of grief, all depend upon the voice for their effect upon the character and the heart. A bad talker is as great a bore as a bad singer or a bad reader. Indeed, to be charming in conversation implies a perfect knowledge of the rare and difficult art of reading. I call it rare and difficult, not only from the nature of the art itself, but also from the great lack of competent teachers. There are a thousand good teachers of the art of singing, where there is *one* of the art of reading. The teachers of *elocution* are generally decayed actors or professors, who are worse than incompetent, for they, in nine cases out of ten, get their pupils into pedantic, affected, and unnatural habits, which are a thousand times worse than the natural awkwardness. The best advice I can give a lady on this subject is—unless she knows a teacher who has an exquisite voice and style—to practise herself in reading aloud, and training her voice to express the most happy and delightful ideas by soft and appropriate tones. She may think herself happy if she acquires perfection in this exquisite art by two years of unwearied pains and study. And she may be sure that the accomplishment is cheaply bought at whatever expense.

CHAPTER XVII

BEAUTY OF DEPORTMENT

*I*t is essential that every lady should understand that the most beautiful and well dressed woman will fail to be *charming* unless all her other attractions are set off with a graceful and fascinating deportment. A pretty face may be seen everywhere, beautiful and gorgeous dresses are common enough, but how seldom do we meet with a really beautiful and enchanting demeanor! It was this charm of deportment which suggested to the French cardinal the expression of "the native paradise of angels." The first thing to be said on the art of deportment is, that what is becoming at one age, would be most improper and ridiculous at another. For a young girl, for instance, to sit as grave and stiff as "her grandmother cut in alabaster" would be ridiculous enough, but not so much so, as for an old woman to assume the romping merriment of girlhood. She would deservedly draw only contempt and laughter upon herself.

Not only woman's age must be consulted, but her manners ought to harmonize with her shape and size, and the whole contour of her style. A deportment which would become a short and thick-set woman would never do for one of a tall and slender figure, with a long neck and contracted waist. The woman of larger proportions may safely affect the majestic gait and air; but how absurd it would be for a tall and slender figure to stiffen her joints, throw back her head, and march off with a military air? The character of these light forms corresponds with their resemblances in the vegetable world. The poplar, the willow, and the graceful lily, bend their gentle heads at every passing breeze, and their flexible and tender arms toss in the wind with motions of grace and beauty. Such is the woman of delicate proportions. She must enter a room either with the buoyant step of a young nymph, if youth is her passport to sportiveness; or, if she is advanced nearer the meridian of life, she may glide in with that ease of manner which gives play to all the graceful motions of her undulating form. For her to crane up her neck would change its swan-like bend into the scraggy throat of an ostrich. All her movements should be of an easy and flexible character. Her mode of salutation should be rather a bow than a courtesy, and when she sits, she should model her attitude after the style of half-recumbent ease, rather than according to the rules of the boarding-school governess, who marshal their pupils on their chairs like a file of drilled recruits. The unassuming, easy, graceful air belongs exclusively to the slender beauty, and the moderated majestic mien to a greater *embonpoint*.

But the least affectation or exaggeration in either of these styles would only end in bringing the woman into contempt. The only safety is for a lady to be governed by those infallible ideas of moderated taste and delicacy, in which the sweetest charms of *modesty* are entrenched.

Indeed a modest mien always makes a woman charming. Modesty is to woman what the mantle of green is to nature—its ornament and highest beauty. What a miracle-working charm there is in a blush—what softness and majesty in natural *simplicity*, without which pomp is contemptible, and elegance itself ungraceful.

There can be no doubt that the highest incitement to love is in modesty. So well do wise women of the world know this, that they take infinite pains to learn to wear the semblance of it, with the same tact, and with the same motive, that they array themselves in attractive apparel. They have taken a lesson from Sir Joshua Reynolds, who says "men are like certain animals, who will feed only when there is but little provender, and that got at with difficulty through the bars of a rack; but refuse to touch it when there is an abundance before them." It is certainly important that all women should understand this, and it is no more than fair that they should practise upon it, since men always treat them with disingenuous untruthfulness in this matter. Men may amuse themselves with a noisy, loud-laughing, loquacious girl; it is the quiet, subdued, modest, and seeming bashful deport which is the one that stands the fairest chance of carrying off their hearts.

CHAPTER XVIII

BEAUTY OF DRESS

*T*he great majority of my sex understand the art of dress no further than that "fine feathers make fine birds;" and hence the women dress more or less in bad taste. Washington Irving says, "in all ages the gentle sex have shown a disposition to infringe a little *upon the laws of decorum*, in order to betray a lurking beauty, or an innocent love of finery."

This is certainly stating the thing very modestly; but, seeing Mr. Irving is a bachelor, it is perhaps going as far as he has any right to do in this direction. It is the *"love of finery,"* however, which is the great source of the corruption of female taste in dress. It is this which *loads* "the lovely form of woman" without *adorning* it.

The first thing to be done in instructing a woman to dress well, is to impress upon her that *profusion* is not *grace*. A lady may empty a merchant's counter upon her person, and yet produce no other effect than to give herself the appearance of a porter's baggage-wagon, loaded with all manner of trinkets.

A lady who dresses in such a manner as to attract attention *to her dress* is always badly dressed. A well-chosen dress so harmonizes with the figure and the general natural style of the lady as to leave the dress itself measurably unobserved. The object of dress should be to show off an *elegant woman*, and not an *elegantly dressed woman*. And therefore, in simplicity, and a certain adaptation to your figure and complexion, all the secret of good dressing lies.

But as beauty of form and complexion varies in different women, and is still more various in different ages, so the styles in dress should assume characters corresponding with all these circumstances. Woman may take a lesson on dress from the garments which nature puts on at the various seasons of the year. In the spring of youth, when all is lovely and gay, and the soft green, sparkling in freshness, bedecks the earth, the light and transparent robes, of brilliant colors, may adorn "the limbs of beauty." Especially if the maid possess the airy form of Hebe, a lightly flowing drapery is best suited to show the loveliness of her charms. This simple garb leaves to beauty all her empire. Let no furbelows, no heavy ornaments, load the figure, or distract the attention in its admiration of the lovely outlines.

The young woman of graver mien and more majestic form, should select her apparel with reference to her different style of beauty. Her robes should always be long and more ample than those of her gayer sister. Their substance should be thicker and of a more sober color. White is considered becoming to all characters; but when colors are to be worn, the lady of majestic style should choose the fuller shades of purple, crimson, scarlet, or black.

The best school to teach a woman taste in dress is the Pantheon of ancient Rome. First behold the lovely Hebe; her robes are like the air, her motion is on the zephyr's wing. That may be woman's style until she is twenty. Then comes the beautiful Diana. The chaste dignity of womanhood and intelligence pervades the whole form, and the very drapery which enfolds it, harmonizes with the modest elegance, the buoyant strength of ripened health, which give elasticity and grace to every limb. That is woman from twenty to thirty. Then comes Juno or Minerva, standing forth in the combined power of beauty and wisdom. "At this period she gradually lays aside the flowers of youth, and arrays herself in the majesty of sobriety, or in the sober beauty of simplicity. Long ought to be the reign of this commanding epoch of woman's age, for from thirty to fifty she may most respectably maintain her station on the throne of matron excellence," and still be lawfully admired as a beautiful woman. But beyond this age, it becomes her to lay aside all such pretensions, and, by her "mantle of grey," gracefully acknowledge her entrance into the "vale of years." What can be more disgusting than a painted and bepowdered old woman, just "trembling on the brink of the grave, and yet a candidate for the flattery of men?"

Not only is it true that there is a propriety in adapting a lady's dress to the different seasons of her life, and the peculiar character of her figure, but there is a *very great propriety* in adapting the *costliness* of her dress to her pecuniary position in life. I know that in America all artificial distinctions of classes are happily laid aside; but the *necessities* which attach to pecuniary disabilities are not, and never can be overcome. Though it may be the right of every woman to dress as expensively as she can afford, yet is it good taste, is it consistent with her own self-respect, for the wife, or the daughter of a poor man

to dress expensively, and imitate all the wasteful extrava-
gances of the rich? Let every such woman be forewarned
that she cannot do it without drawing upon herself the
inevitable suspicion that must cause a husband and a
father to blush, even though the purple tinge never visits
her own cheek. Though she may be innocent, it is still
bad taste to effect expenditures beyond her known means
or income. There is a fitness, and an inexpressible charm,
in the sight of a woman who adapts her neat and modest
attire to the circumstances of her life.

CHAPTER XIX

BEAUTY OF ORNAMENTS

O n this subject, the rule is, as laid down by a time-honored maxim, that "beauty unadorned, is adorned the most." As a general remark, we may say that to a beautiful woman ornaments are unnecessary, and to one who is not beautiful, they are unavailing. But still, as gems and ornaments are handsome in themselves, a beautiful young woman, "if she chooses to share her empire with the jeweller and florist, may, not inelegantly, decorate her neck, arms and head with something like a string of pearls and a band of flowers."

A young lady, however, of fair complexion and slender figure can find no adornment in gems, as they are too heavy for her style of beauty. Her ornaments can rarely exceed the natural or artificial flowers of the most delicate kind—such as the violet, the snow-drop, the myrtle, the primrose, or the lily of the valley. The garments of a young beauty of this style should be of white, or of the most tender shades of green, pink, blue and lilac. These, when judiciously selected, or mingled, array the graceful wearer like another Iris, "breathing youth and loveliness." As a general thing all ornaments detract from the exceeding charms of such beauty.

All ornaments for the head are, to say the least, a dangerous experiment. If a lady's hair is very beautiful and abundant, it will be difficult to select an ornament that can add anything to its charms; and if it is coarse and harsh, and of a bad color, she surely will not commit the blunder of attracting attention to it by gems and ornaments. So, if her neck and bosom be of a pearly whiteness, and fashioned after "nature's most enchanting mould," what ornament can add to its fascination? And if they are naturally dingy and brown, and lack the delicate outline of symmetrical beauty, why should she needlessly attract attention to her deformity by a sparkling necklace, or a string of pearls!

So too of her hands; if the fingers are long and bony, or lack the delicate taper and "pearl-tipped nails," why will she attract all eyes to her misfortune, with the glitter of rings and diamonds? A single diamond on a beautiful hand, or some light and rich bracelet on an arm which is charming enough to bear constant inspection, may not be inappropriate; but a profusion of these ornaments is always in bad taste, and a sure sign of vulgarity, or of deficient education.

I have, however, known some artful belles who contrived quite successfully to deceive the men with regard to their incurably dingy necks and bosoms, by covering the whole with a soft, white lace shirt, over which was placed a necklace of beautiful pearls, leaving upon the eye of the beholder the most enchanting ideas of what was hid beneath. A lady who has ugly arms may employ the same art, by the use of long sleeves, of the whitest and finest material, with a neat cuff, made to fit close to the wrist, and fastened with some rich jewel. But these are delicate arts, and require great discrimination and good taste to be used successfully.

Let every woman be taught to know that the danger ever lies in the use of *too many*, rather than in *too few* ornaments.

CHAPTER XX

IMPORTANCE OF HAIR

AS AN ORNAMENT

Without a fine head of hair no woman can be really beautiful. A combination of perfect features, united in one person, would all go for naught without that *crowning* excellence of beautiful hair. Take the handsomest woman that ever lived—one with the finest eyes, a perfect nose, an expanded forehead, a charming face, and a pair of lips that beat the ripest and reddest cherries of summer—and shave her head, and what a fright would she be! The dogs would bark at, and run from her in the street.

The same thing is true of man. How like a fool or a ruffian do the noblest masculine features appear if the hair of the head is bad? And, on the other hand, the most defective features are more than half redeemed by a fine head of hair. Many a dandy, who has scarcely brains enough or courage enough to catch a sheep, has enslaved the hearts of a hundred girls with his Hyperion locks.

We ought, then, to be constantly impressed with the importance of hair as a chief ornament in beauty. It is every person's business to be informed of the means of developing and preserving a luxurious growth of this handmaid of human charms.

And it is in the power of almost every person to have a good head of hair. But, by many, such a gift can be enjoyed only by great pains and constant attention to the laws of its growth and preservation. Hair left to take care of itself will revenge itself by making its possessor either common looking, or a monster of ugliness. Let the woman who is ambitious to be beautiful not forget this. I have known women, who had scarcely another charm to commend them, to carry off scores of hearts by a bountiful and beautiful head of hair.

CHAPTER XXI

HOW TO OBTAIN

A GOOD HEAD OF HAIR

*T*he foundation of a good head of hair ought undoubtedly to be laid in infancy. At this tender age, and through all the years of childhood, it should be worn short, be frequently cut, and never allowed to go a day without a thorough brushing. It should also, every morning, be washed at the roots with cold water. A damp sponge, rubbed thoroughly upon the scalp, will be sufficient. The practice of combing the heads of children too frequently with a fine tooth comb is a bad one, as the points of the teeth are quite sure to scratch and irritate the scalp, and are almost sure to produce scurf or dandruff. Indeed, these rules, except as to the *length* of the hair, are quite as applicable to adults as to children. The ladies of my acquaintance, who have been most celebrated for the beauty of their hair, usually made a practice of thoroughly cleansing its roots every morning with the damp sponge. Nor would they venture to neglect the frequent use of the brush. Indeed, the coarsest, most refractory, and snarly locks can be subdued, and made comparatively soft and glossy by the use of the brush alone. Constant *brushing* is the first rule to subdue coarse and brittle hair. And the morning is the best time for an extended application of the brush, because the hair is naturally more supple then than at any other time. This practice, thoroughly persevered in, will gradually tame down the porcupine head, unless there is some scurfy disease of the scalp, in which case the following wash will be found a quite sure remedy:—

Salts of tartar	3 drachms.
Tincture of cantharides	15 drops.
Spirits of camphor	15 drops.
Lemon juice	½ pint.

In preparing this wash, the salts should be dissolved in the lemon juice, till the effervescence ceases, and then add the other ingredients; and, after letting the whole remain exposed to the air for half an hour, it may be perfumed and bottled for use. This is one of the best and most harmless washes for the hair I have ever known. I am certain that a lady or gentleman has but to try it to be convinced of its efficacy. But let me impress upon you the importance of *brushing* as a cardinal means of beautifying the hair. *Brush* not *one* minute, but *ten*—not once a day, but two, or three, or four times a day.

Two brushes are indispensable for the toilet—one for the rough use of cleaning the hair, and the other for polishing it. A black brush should be used for the former, and a white one for the latter. Ladies need not be told that washing spoils brushes. The way to clean them is to rub them thoroughly with bran, which removes all the grease, and leaves the bristles stiff and firm as ever. When the bristles of a brush become too limber for use, they may be hardened again by dipping them in one part of spirits of ammonia, and two of water. This will also thoroughly cleanse them from all greasy substances.

CHAPTER XXII

TO PREVENT THE HAIR

FROM FALLING OFF

A remedy for weak and falling hair has been sought for by beautiful women, and by men too, with as much avidity as ever the mad enthusiast sought for the philosopher's stone. I have known ladies who did nothing but to hunt recipes for baldness. The knowledge of all their friends, especially if they were physicians, was laid under perpetual contribution for light on the great subject of hair. I knew an old countess in Paris—or who was at least fearfully growing old—who became really a monomaniac on this subject; she used to rattle on about the "bulbs of the hair," the "apex of the hair," and talk as learnedly as a whole college of doctors of the various theories of the nature of the disease and the remedy. Some quack had recommended her to use caustic alkalies of soda or potash—which by the way I have known to be advised by physicians who ought to know better—which completely did the business for her head, for, they not only destroyed the reproductive power, but also the *color* of what hair they left upon her head. So that this unhappy countess was not only hopelessly grey, but she was growing balder day by day, notwithstanding half a bushel of recipes which she had wrung from the skill of a hundred doctors.

It is well known that Baron Dupuytren obtained a world-wide fame for a pomade which actually overcame the evil of baldness in thousands of cases where it was applied. A celebrated physician in London gave to an intimate friend of mine the following recipe which he assured her was really the famous pomade of Baron Dupuytren. My friend found such advantage in its use that I was induced to copy it, and add it to my cabinet of curious recipes.

> Boxwood shavings . . 6 oz.
> Proof spirit . . . . . . 12 oz.
> Spirits of rosemary . . 2 oz.
> Spirits of nutmegs . . . ½ oz.

The boxwood shavings should be left to steep in the spirits, at a temperature of 60 degrees, for fourteen days, and then the liquid should be strained off, and the other ingredients mixed. The scalp to be thoroughly washed, or rubbed with this every night and morning.

A vulgar notion prevails that shaving the head once or twice is a good thing to overcome the tendency towards falling hair. But it is a fatal error, which stands a fair chance of producing incurable baldness; as the hair is apt to be killed by being cut so near the roots. I knew a beautiful lady at Madrid who suffered in this way. I advise everybody who has weak hair to avoid wearing nightcaps, and to adopt in their place a net-cap, with coarse meshes, which will allow the heat of the head to pass freely off.

CHAPTER XXIII

TO PREVENT THE HAIR

FROM TURNING GREY

*N*o woman must rely on compounds and powders to prevent her hair from turning grey. Temperance, moderation in all things, and frequent washings with pure, cold water are the best recipes I can give her to prevent her hair from becoming prematurely grey. It is certain that perpetual care, great anxiety, or prolonged grief will hasten white hairs. History has made us familiar with instances where sudden passion, or grief, or fright, have turned the head instantly grey. Sickness, we know, often does it. But, so far as I know, physiologists have failed to explain the reason of this change. We know that the hair is a hollow tube, containing a fluid which gives it its color—that red hair is occasioned by a red fluid, and so all the varieties of color are owing to the variety of the color of this fluid. Nothing therefore can prevent the hair from turning white but the avoidance of all the causes which produce premature old age, or occasion local obstruction and disease of the hair itself. I have reason to believe that the injudicious use of the curling-irons, long kept up, will hasten this disease. The unnatural heat destroys the animal nature of the hair, and is liable to produce a disease of its coloring fluid.

An old and retired actress with whom I had met at Gibraltar, and who had a fine head of hair, far better preserved than the rest of her charms, was confident that she had warded off the approach of grey hair by using the following preparation whenever she dressed her head.

Oxide of bismuth . . 4 drs.
Spermaceti . . . . . . 4 drs.
Pure hog's lard . . . 4 oz.

The lard and spermaceti should be melted together, and when they begin to cool stir in the bismuth. It may be perfumed to your liking.

CHAPTER XXIV

HOW TO SOFTEN AND

BEAUTIFY THE HAIR

*T*here is no greater mistake than the profuse use of greases for the purpose of softening the hair. They obstruct the pores, the free action of which is so necessary for the health of the hair. No substance should be employed which cannot be readily absorbed by the vessels. These preparations make the hair dry and harsh, unless perpetually loaded with an offensive and disgusting amount of grease.

There was a celebrated beauty at Munich who had one of the handsomest heads of hair I ever beheld, and she used regularly to wash her head every morning with the following:

Beat up the white of four eggs into a froth, and rub that thoroughly in close to the roots of the hair. Leave it to dry on. Then wash the head and hair clean with a mixture of equal parts of rum and rose-water.

This will be found one of the best cleansers and brighteners of the hair that was ever used.

There is a celebrated wash called "Honey Water" known to fashionable ladies all over Europe, which is made as follows:

Essence of Ambergris	. .	1 dr.
" Musk	. . . .	1 dr.
" Bergamot	. .	2 drs.
Oil of Cloves	. . . . .	15 drops.
Orange-flower water	. . .	4 oz.
Spirits of wine	. . . . . .	5 oz.
Distilled water	. . . . . .	4 oz.

All these ingredients should be mixed together, and left about fourteen days, then the whole to be filtered through porous paper, and bottled for use.

This is a good hair-wash and an excellent perfume.

But let the man or woman who is ambitious to have handsome hair, forget not that frequent and thorough *brushing* is worth all the oils and pomades that were ever invented.

CHAPTER XXV

TO REMOVE SUPERFLUOUS HAIR

*I*t sometimes happens that feminine beauty is a little marred by an unfeminine growth of hair on the upper lip, or on the neck and arms, and sometimes on the chin. I have known several unfortunate ladies to produce ulcers and dangerous sores by compounds which they used for the purpose of removing these blemishes. Caustic preparations of lime, arsenic, and potash have been used for this purpose with the above results.

But the following safe method has been used with perfect success:

Spread on a piece of leather equal parts of galbanum and pitch plaster, and lay it on the culprit hairs as smoothly as possible, and then, after letting it remain about three minutes, pull it off suddenly, and it will be quite sure to bring out the hairs by the roots, and they will not grow again. The pain of this operation is much less than the cauterizing remedy, and is, besides, more successful. I have seen poor victims sit all day pulling these aggressive hairs with tweezers, which is a fruitless task, for they almost invariably break off the hair at the neck, instead of pulling it out by the roots. But the most ridiculous mistake which women make in this business is removing the superfluous hair with a razor, for that promotes the unnatural growth, and, even though the shaving were done every day, the blue or black roots of the hair show further than the hair itself.

CHAPTER XXVI

HOW TO COLOR GREY HAIR

A great many compounds, which are of a character most destructive to the hair, are sold in the shape of hair-dyes, against which ladies cannot be too frequently warned. These, for the most part, are composed of such things as poisonous mineral acids, nitrate and oxide of silver, caustic alkalies, lime, litharge and arsenic. The way these *color* the hair is simply by *burning* it, and they are very liable to produce a disease of the hair which increases ten-fold the speed of growing grey. One patent hair-dye was proved on analysis to be a preparation of hydrophosphuret of ammonia, a most filthy ingredient, which, besides its villainous smell, would cause immediate suffocation if inhaled by the lungs. All these patent compounds rot the hair, if they do no greater mischief.

An old physician and chemist at Lisbon gave a charming Parisian lady of my acquaintance, whose hair was turning grey, on one side of her head after a severe sickness, a recipe for a hair-dye which proved to be of astonishing efficacy in coloring the faded hair a beautiful and natural black. The following is the recipe for making it:

Gallic acid . . . . 10 grs.
Acetic acid . . . . 1 oz.
Tincture of sesqui-chloride of iron . . 1 oz.

Dissolve the gallic acid in the tincture of sesqui-chloride of iron, and then add the acetic acid. Before using this preparation, the hair should be thoroughly washed with soap and water. A great and desirable peculiarity of this dye, is that it can be so applied as to color the hair either *black* or the lighter shade of brown. If *black* is the color desired, the preparation should be applied while the hair is moist, and for *brown* it should not be used till the hair is perfectly dry. The way to apply the compound is to dip the points of a fine tooth comb into it until the interstices are filled with the fluid, then gently draw the comb through the hair, commencing at the roots, till the dye has perceptibly taken effect. When the hair is entirely dry, oil and brush it as usual.

CHAPTER XXVII

HABITS WHICH DESTROY

BEAUTIFUL HAIR

The habit of frequently shampooing the hair, or washing it with soap and water, is destructive to its beauty. Soap, if often used, will be likely to change the color of the hair to a faded yellowish hue, even if it does not produce a greater misfortune. The best way to remove dust, or the effects of an indiscreet use of oils or pomades from the hair is to give it a thorough brushing. Or a small quantity of white soap may be dissolved in spirits of wine, and used without deleterious effects. But, by all means, shun strong soap, and such alkaline lyes as are used in shampooing; for these lyes are capable of dissolving the hair if long left in them, and their use is invariably deleterious. As a general thing, set down all the patent nostrums puffed in newspapers as useless, if they are not positively hurtful. Even if we were sure that they are scientifically compounded, we may be certain that they are made of the poorest and cheapest qualities of materials. But since we know that they are almost invariably mixed by quacks and imposters, it seems strange that any lady will trust so great and indispensable a charm as that of her hair to the mercies of irresponsible ignorance and avarice.

Washing the hair even with cold water and leaving it to dry in curls, as is the custom of some, after the example of Lord Byron, renders it harsh and coarse. Whenever the hair is washed it should be thoroughly dried with towels, and then be well brushed.

CHAPTER XXVIII

BLEMISHES TO BEAUTY

There are a great many accidental blemishes to beauty, such as pimples, black specks, freckles, tan, and yellow spots, which may be removed by proper remedies faithfully applied.

To Remove Pimples

There are many kinds of pimples, some of which partake almost of the nature of ulcers, which require medical treatment; but the small red pimple, which is most common, may be removed by applying the following twice a day:

Sulphur water	1 oz.
Acetated liquor of ammonia	¼ oz.
Liquor of potassa	1 gr.
White wine vinegar	2 oz.
Distilled water	2 oz.

These pimples are sometimes cured by frequent washing in warm water, and prolonged friction with a coarse towel. The cause of these pimples is obstruction of the skin and imperfect circulation.

To Remove Black Specks or "Fleshworms"

Sometimes little black specks appear about the base of the nose, or on the forehead, or in the hollow of the chin, which are called "fleshworms," and are occasioned by coagulated lymph that obstructs the pores of the skin. They may be squeezed out by pressing the skin, and ignorant people suppose them to be little worms. They are permanently removed by washing with warm water, and severe friction with a towel, and then applying a little of the following preparation:

> Liquor of potassa . . 1 oz.
> Cologne . . . . 2 oz.
> White brandy . . . . 4 oz.

The warm water and friction alone are sometimes sufficient.

To Remove Freckles

The most celebrated compound ever used for the removal of freckles was called *Unction de Maintenon*, after the celebrated Madame de Maintenon, mistress and wife of Louis XIV. It is made as follows:

> Venice soap . . . . 1 oz.
> Lemon juice . . . . ½ oz.
> Oil of bitter almonds . . . . ¼ oz.
> Deliquidated oil of tartar . . ¼ oz.
> Oil of rhodium . . . . . . 3 drops.

First dissolve the soap in the lemon juice, then add the two oils, and place the whole in the sun till it acquires the consistence of ointment, and then add the oil of rhodium. Anoint the freckly face at night with this unction, and wash in the morning with pure water, or if convenient, with a mixture of elder-flower and rose-water.

To Remove Tan

An excellent wash to remove tan is called *Crême de l'Enclos*, and is thus made:

New milk . . . . . ½ pint.
Lemon juice . . . ¼ oz.
White brandy . . ½ oz.

Boil the whole, and skim it clear from all scum. Use it night and morning.

A famous preparation with the Spanish ladies for removing the effects of the sun and making the complexion bright, is composed simply of equal parts of lemon juice and the white of eggs. The whole is beat together in a varnished earthen pot, and set over a slow fire, and stirred with a wooden spoon till it acquires the consistence of soft pomatum. This compound is called *Pommade de Seville*. If the face is well washed with rice-water before it is applied, it will remove freckles, and give a fine lustre to the complexion.

To Cure Chapped Lips

A certain cure for chapped lips, used by the French ladies, is called *Baume à l'Antique* and is thus made.

Oil of roses . . 4 oz.
White wax . . . 1 oz.
Spermaceti . . . ½ oz.

They should be melted in a glass vessel, and stirred with a wooden spoon till thoroughly mixed, and then poured into a glass or china cup for use.

To Remove Yellow Spots

Sometimes yellow spots of various sizes appear under the skin of the neck and face, and prove the most annoying blemishes to beauty. I have known them to be effectually removed by rubbing them with the flour of sulphur until they disappeared. The following wash is also a safe remedy—

> Strong sulphur water . . 1 oz.
> Lemon juice . . . . . . ¼ oz.
> Cinnamon water . . . . 1 dra.

Wash with this three or four times a day. Sometimes these spots indicate a difficulty in the stomach which may require medical advice.

To Remove and Prevent Wrinkles

There is a curious recipe called *Aura and Cephalus* which is of Grecian origin, as its name would indicate, and is said to have been most efficacious in removing and preventing premature wrinkles from the faces of the Athenian ladies.

Put some powder of best myrrh upon an iron plate, sufficiently heated to melt the gum gently, and when it liquifies, cover your head with a napkin, and hold your face over the myrrh at a proper distance to receive the fumes without inconvenience. I will observe, however, that if this experiment produces any symptoms of headache, it better be discontinued at once.

But an easy and natural way of warding off wrinkles is frequent ablution, followed by prolonged friction with a dry napkin. If a lady is a little advanced towards the period when wrinkles are naturally expected to make their appearance, she should use tepid water instead of cold, in her ablutions.

To Remove Stains or Spots From Silk

If a lady has the misfortune to stain a silk dress, the following preparation will remove the stain without injuring the silk.

Take five ounces of soft water and six ounces of alum well pounded; boil the mixture for a short time, then pour it in a vessel to cool. Previous to using it, it must be made warm, when the stained part may be washed with it and left to dry.

To Remove Grease From Silks

Wash the soiled part with ether, and the grease will disappear.

HINTS TO GENTLEMEN

ON THE ART OF FASCINATING

FIFTY RULES

IN THE ART OF

FASCINATING

I *expect* to win the gratitude of the whole masculine gender by these rules of the ART OF FASCINATING. It used to be supposed that this art belonged exclusively to my sex; but that was a vulgar error, which the sharp practice of the men has long since exploded. And it is now well established that gentlemen spend a great deal more time in inventing ways and means to entrap women and get them in love with them, than women do in trying to win the hearts of gentlemen. Love making, indeed, seems to be the "being's end and aim" of man. He appears to think that he was born for no other purpose, and he devotes himself to the business with a zeal and an enthusiasm highly honorable to his exalted genius, and to the immortal station he claims for himself of being the *lord of creation*.

To become a proficient in the art of fascinating, therefore, is not merely an *accomplishment* and a *pastime* but it is a *duty* which he may not neglect without incurring the gravest censure of mankind. In entering upon the study of this great and important art, to start correctly, he must take it for granted that women are not only very poor judges of men, but that they absolutely prefer fops, fools, and triflers, to men of sense and character. If, how-ever, the student has doubts on this subject he had better refer to certain learned authorities which will not fail to establish his mind in the right premises. Mackenzie says "women have a predilection for frivolous men." One of the most learned of the British Essayists says, "when we see a fellow loud and talkative, full of insipid life and laughter, we may venture to pronounce him a female fa-vorite." Mr. Burke tells you that "the character which generally passes for *agreeable* with the women is made up of civility and falsehood." And if poets were of any au-thority in this high art, I might refer to Dryden who sings—

> *"Our thoughtless sex is caught by outward form*
> *And empty noise—and* loves itself in man."

If these learned authorities fail to satisfy the mind of my pupils, I shall beg to refer them to the works of Sir Walter Raleigh and Lord Chesterfield, who are very co-pious on this subject. But as they progress in the experi-mental part of the art, they will learn to rely less on authorities, and trust more to their own experience and skill. Indeed I have seldom met with a man who did not consider himself, in his way, such a proficient in this sub-lime art that it may be wasting time to dwell at all upon the subject of *authorities*.

Rule the First

Set it down, then, that the women prefer *triflers* to men of *sense*, and when you wish to make one of the sex tre-mendously in love with you, you will of course make yourself as big a fool as possible, in order to ensure the most speedy and triumphant success. You will do this not only because women prefer such characters, but you will also consider that so little do the most sensible and fascinating women know of their own power, that, Nero-like, they will only stop to catch flies and gnats.

Your hope of complete success, then, lies in your ability to be a coxcomb, who has no earthly recommendation but his face, his coat, and his impudence. To acquire pleasing and fascinating manners you will do well to spend about half of your time between the curling-irons and the looking-glass, so as to become the paragon described by Mr. Tennyson.

> *"Oiled and curled like an Assyrian bull,*
> *Smelling of musk and insolence."*

Rule the Second

You will make an immense hit with the ladies by pretending to be no admirer of any particular woman, but a professed adorer and slave of the whole sex; a thing which you can easily show by staring insultingly at every pretty woman you meet. This will also be following the analogy of nature, as we know that fleas and other disgusting insects molest those who have the tenderest skins and fairest complexions, just as the human flesh-flies haunt the fairer part of creation. Then, as you are not a *particular*, but only a *general* lover, the ladies will regard it as a safe business to receive the fractional part of your heart which might belong to them, just as a popular notion prevails that homeopathic doses of medicine are *harmless,* to say the least.

Rule the Third

You will do well to boast that you have no higher ambition in life than merely to render yourself *agreeable to the ladies.* This will at once impress them with profound respect for the magnitude of your ambition, and the majesty of your genius. Every woman will be crazy to marry a man of such splendid prospects; and the whole sex will be most happy to avail themselves of the services of so amiable and useful a gentleman. But let me caution you not to give the slightest heed to those cast-iron, sneering kind of men who out of jealousy, will say that you were framed by nature to be a woman's fool, and who will further seek to annoy you by saying that the ladies change their lackey-lovers as often as they do their bonnets, because they soon get tired of them.

Rule the Fourth

If you can affect effeminacy and a lisping softness in your speech it will go a great way towards winning the confidence and esteem of a sensible and lovely woman. Let your conversation never rise out of the level of balls, parties, fashions and the opera. The *opera* will be not only a pleasing but an appropriate theme for you, as it will associate you, in the lady's mind, with the charming subject of *music*, reminding her that quavers and unmeaning words are always *softer* than its more manly parts.

Rule the Fifth

By all means wear jewelry; if you have it not of your own, borrow it, or get it some other way, for you must be sure that you go not into the presence of any woman, whose good opinion is worth having, without being loaded with jewelry. An immense breast-pin, either of diamonds or paste, with two rings on each hand and a heavy fob chain, twelve inches long, will be sufficient to prove that you are a man of substantial good sense, and that you are the possessor of a heart which is worthy of the confidence and admiration of any woman.

Rule the Sixth

Remember that faint heart never won fair lady yet, and that, therefore, you must push your suit with the determination and vehemence of an army of soldiers storming a fort. Women like men of courage, therefore you should entertain the lady you would win with a narration of the number of men you have knocked down, at balls and bar-rooms, who had the temerity to cross your path. Be sure that you always make yourself the hero of some scrape, for, notwithstanding the ladies will readily know that you are telling lies all the time, yet you show that you have a *taste* for fighting, and that you really possess all the attributes of a hero but the more brutal part of it—*courage*.

Rule the Seventh

Remember that we do not like men for the merit we may discover in them, so much as for that they can find in us; therefore be sure that no man out-fawns you in the attentions paid to the woman of your choice. Let your compliments be of so marked a character that there can be no mistaking them. For instance, you may ask her if she is always particular to shut her eyes on retiring to bed? She will ask *why*? And you will answer, *Because if you do not, I fear that the brightness of your eyes will burn holes in the blanket, or set the house afire!* This kind of compliment is of the most delicate nature, and will be certain to impress the lady, especially if she is a person of sense, with the sincerity and purity of your intentions.

Rule the Eighth

You cannot be too attentive to your dress. You should never approach a lady except when dressed so as to look precisely as though a tailor had made you not more than fifteen minutes before. Be careful that your figure is consulted in the color and fit of your garments. If you are tall and lank, wear nothing but black, that you may "appear like a stick of black sealing-wax," which will impress the ladies with an idea of the adhesive quality of your nature. If you are short and dumpy, and "better made for rolling than for running," you will look particularly handsome in light or grey clothes, which will greatly enhance your fine rotundity. If your legs are small and crooked, do not fail to have your pants cut to fit a little tighter than your skin, as this will show to great advantage the delicacy of your proportions, while, at the same time, it will familiarize a lady's eye to the sight of those disgusting spiders, which, otherwise, might cause great mischief by sudden frights. If you are wise, you will not fail to impress upon a lady's mind the idea that you are a great deal more particular about your *clothes* than your *mind,* for your mind, being always out of sight, can never offend her taste, whereas your clothes are constantly before her eyes.

Rule the Ninth

On being introduced to a lady you will immediately inform her that you consider that the proper study of mankind is *woman,* and that Pope was therefore wrong when he asserted it to be *man.* You will proceed to say that you have made the sex your study so long that you find it impossible to withdraw your mind from a constant inspection of everything a lady says and does. This she will receive as a great compliment paid to her sex, while it will be particularly pleasing to her to know that she has such a competent and vigilant spy upon all her actions.

Rule the Tenth

If you are invited to dine, go at least an hour, or an hour and a half before the time, for then the lady will be sure *never to forget you*, as the attentive and polite gentleman who allowed her neither time to dress, nor to superintend her dinner. Or, if it is not convenient to go so long beforehand, you had best not go till twenty minutes, or half an hour after the time, and so keep the dinner waiting, for this will get the lady in the habit of thinking of you when you are absent, which is a great point gained in the progress of love. But, under no circumstances must you arrive at the place about five or ten minutes before the dinner hour, for should you do so, the lady will be reminded of the vulgar showman, who cries—"Be in time, be in time—just going to begin—be in time."

Rule the Eleventh

Much depends on your conduct at the table; for ladies are very observant of all such little affairs. To give one a good idea of your gentility, take your napkin and tie it round your neck as a "bib," turn up your coat sleeves, and fall to, without paying any attention to the lady who sits next you, for ladies like not to be disturbed at meals. To show that you relish your food, let your mastication be quite audible, and when you drink to a lady, say "here's luck," smack your lips, and cry "ha!" Nothing gives a lady a more exalted idea of a man than to see that he is fond of good eating and drinking.

Rule the Twelfth

When you call upon a lady be sure that you say something smart, and make some local hit applicable to herself. For instance, if you perceive that she has a *cough,* you can say that you are sorry to hear that, as you fear it may lead to a *coffin.* Some such sublime joke as this will be sure to obtain you a favorable reception. Or you can entertain her, to a remarkable degree, by relating the number of your female friends who have died of consumption within a year, and you can wind up by quoting the following words of Moore:

> *"I never had a dear gazelle*
> *To glad me with its mild blue eye,*
> *But when it came to know me well*
> *And love me, it was sure to die."*

This will make her particularly anxious to be considered one of your "female friends."

Rule the Thirteenth

If you invite a lady to go to the theatre, neglect not to leave her, and go out to drink with your male friends between each act, as this will show her that you have confidence that she can protect herself; and if you can fall asleep during the play, it will be a great thing for you, as it will show that you are too much interested in her to take any interest in the play; and, besides, she has the sweet privilege of imagining that you are dreaming of her.

Nothing so fascinates a woman as to know that a gentle-man dreams about her. Hence you will do well to always pretend that you dreamed of her, whether you did or not. No matter if she understands your falsehood, as she will be quite sure to do, for still she cannot help being flat-tered that you think so much of her that you will tell her falsehoods to please her.

Rule the Fourteenth

It will be greatly to your advantage to entertain the lady you would win with an account of the number of women who are in love with you, and of the decided advances which they have made to *you*; for this will not only prove that you are a great favorite with the ladies, and a man of true honor, but it will convince her that she may have the honor of being enrolled in the same list, and of being praised in the same way, in the presence of your other female friends. This will greatly delight her, and you need not be surprised if she testifies her admiration of your character by throwing her arms around your neck on the spot. And if afterwards you should hear of her having said that you *ought to be hanged,* you will, of course, understand that she wants to use her own lovely arms for the *halter.*

Rule the Fifteenth

One of the most direct and sure ways to fascinate a lady, is to excite in her heart a spirit of rivalry, through jeal-ousy. A common way of doing this is to get the daguerreo-types of your father's *cook* and *chambermaid*, and take them to your lady-love, and tell her that they are the like-nesses of two very rich and highly respectable ladies who have for a long time persecuted you with their affections, and at last have had the indelicacy to send you their pictures, without any solicitation on your part whatever. This story will readily be believed, as everybody knows that *rich and respectable* ladies are in the habit of doing just such things, and it will certainly convince any lady that you are a prize worth having, especially as she foresees that she would have the pleasure of having her home filled with a cabinet of strange women's faces, which she could exhibit as the proud savage does the scalps her husband has taken from the heads of his enemies.

Rule the Sixteenth

If a lady you admire happens to make the acquaintance of some gentleman of superior attainments and position to yourself, make yourself as boorish to him as possible, whenever you meet him in her company, for this will be sure to increase her admiration of *you*, and cause her to despise *him*. And then, the moment he leaves, you will be able to demolish him entirely by assailing his character —making him out a rascal, a roué and a libertine, of the very blackest dye; and fail not to believe that the blacker you paint him, the whiter you will look yourself. This course cannot fail to bring her to her senses, and convince her what a fool she has made of herself by taking such a ruffian and scoundrel for a gentleman. And then she will admire you beyond description as the *discoverer* of his villainy, especially as she will clearly perceive the motives you had for the exercise of such an extraordinary sagacity. By this course you will open to her mind a vein of certain commendable traits of character possessed in an eminent degree by yourself, and to which she might otherwise have forever remained a stranger.

Rule the Seventeenth

If you have not learning, by all means *pretend* to have it, for this will give a lady, and all her friends, an opportunity of laughing at you, which will make you a most agreeable and amusing fellow in her estimation. But, if, on the other hand, you really possess some little learning, do not fail to show it off on all occasions. If a lady does not know a word of French, you will, of course, intersperse your conversation plentifully with words from that language. You may ask her if she has ever read *"Les Egarements du Cœur?"* She will stare at you to see if you are mad, and you will have the pleasure of relieving her alarm by telling her it is the name of a French book, the English of which is "The Wanderings of the Heart," and which you believe has never been translated into our language. She will think you really a charming man for having relieved the distressing anxiety which you had created. Now you can not only talk in English on the delightful subject of *hearts*, but, having given her a taste of French, you can proceed to give her a useful and pleasing lesson in that language. You may tell her that you learned it very easily, that the words are very simple, and you can prove yourself by informing her that the French word for fool is *folle*, and for ass, is *âne*, that the masculine article a, is *un*, and that *et* means and, that therefore *un folle et un âne* means *a fool and an ass*. If there is no one by to correct your bad French, you will get credit for being a great scholar, while the lady will be profoundly impressed with the beauty and *propriety* of your first lesson in French, and she will be sure never to forget *you* as long as she remembers *it*.

Rule the Eighteenth

It will be a masterly stroke of policy for you to pretend to be an *atheist*, and to scoff at every idea of religion; for, if you have no respect for your Maker, nor for anything that mankind holds sacred, it will satisfy any intelligent and reflecting lady that you will have all the more respect and love to bestow upon her.

Rule the Nineteenth

You ought to know that there are four things which always possess more or less interest to a lady—a parrot, a peacock, a monkey, and a man; and the nearer you can come to uniting all these about equally in your own character, the more will you be loved. This is also a cheap and excellent recipe for making a dandy—a creature which is always an object of admiration and esteem to the ladies.

Rule the Twentieth

As *heels* are of more importance to men than *heads*, you will, of course, spend all of your earlier days in learning to dance, and when you are perfected in the art, you cannot do better than spend the rest of your time in dancing. Fail not to convince a lady that your *real existence* is in the ball-room, and that during all the intervening time your godlike faculties are simply taking their natural sleep. You must not dance as a mere pastime and as an occasional amusement, but you must devote yourself to it as a business and a religion

"For which you wish to live or dare to die."

Dance with all the might of your body, and all the fire of your soul, in order that you may shake all melancholy out of your liver; and you need not restrain yourself with the apprehension that any lady will have the least fear that the violence of your movements will ever shake anything out of your brains.

Rule the Twenty-first

Nothing so readily fascinates a lady as *wit*; but as this is a very rare thing, and only one in ten thousand really possess it, the best you can do is, *affect* it—that is, you can try to be witty, and even if you should fail, the lady's laughter will testify how much she is delighted at your effort. Puns are always delightful, and you must not forget those only are *good* which are decidedly *bad*, a fact which is all in your favor. Should you hear a lady tell her servant to *bring up* the dinner, a delicate piece of wit would be to affect great astonishment, and exclaim, *"bring up the dinner!* pray tell me, madam, has your servant *swallowed* the dinner?"* Or you can make a misstep, and bump your head against hers, if you dare risk your own in such a collision and say, "Beg pardon, but you know *two heads are better than one;"* and even if you should happen to break a shell side-comb, and give her a headache for a day, she will forgive it because of the manliness and delicacy of your wit. Or you might contrive to kick her leg with the toe of your boot, until she cries out with pain, which will give you a chance to defend yourself by declaring that she has "no right to complain, as it was perfectly *leg*-al." Only treat a lady with such refined and charming wit as this, and she will be sure to betray the

tenderest regard for you, by affectionately wishing you
were in "Abraham's bosom."

Rule the Twenty-second

Should you invite a lady out to supper, you must, by all
means, order three times as much of expensive dishes as
it will be possible for you to eat, as this will show her that
you have a generous disregard of money, and would just
as soon waste it, as spend it economically, which will convince her that your wife will never want for money, *i.e.*
if you have any yourself.

If it is not convenient to be so expensive, take the other
extreme, and be as mean as possible. Contemn all dishes,
that cost over fifteen cents, as being out of season or as
unhealthy; and *all wines* you are to denounce as vile
drugs, which you will neither drink yourself nor offer to
those whom you respect. Then order ale for two, which,
as she will probably not drink of it, you will have all to
yourself; and, as you put the glass to your lips blow off
the froth, or head, and say *"here's to you"*—a compliment
she cannot fail to appreciate and admire.

Rule the Twenty-third

Whenever you call on a lady, speak of having "just come
from the club," and dwell with pride upon the amount of
time you spend there, because all ladies have great faith
in the happy influence of such places as "clubs" upon a
young man, in not only teaching him the polite accomplishments of *chewing* and *drinking*, and a great many
coarser habits, but they get him into the pleasant way of
late hours, and of spending all his leisure time away from
home. There is no sensible lady who will not jump at the

chance of marrying one of these *club-men*, for she knows that she will be relieved of his company nearly all the time, and that she will, furthermore, have the great pleasure of sitting up to welcome him home at the poetical hour of midnight. What a charming prospect for domestic happiness!

Rule the Twenty-fourth

You must do everything in your power to convince a lady that you are, in a modest way, a great admirer of beauty; an excellent way to prove which is, to be always seen, on rainy days, when the streets are muddy, standing at the corners, where most ladies pass, staring at the embarrassments of pedestrian beauty, picking its blushing way through the mud. This is a compliment to the ladies, and a proof of your *modest* and *elevated* admiration of the beautiful, which every respectable woman will duly appreciate. And, by simply reflecting upon the gratitude with which you would see the same delicate attentions paid to your own wife or daughter, you can more fully realize the fascinating excellence of your character.

Rule the Twenty-fifth

Of course you will never allow yourself to sit five minutes by the side of a lady without paying her some respectful and delicate attention, such as taking her handkerchief, and spreading it out on your lap, or leaning affectionately upon her, or throwing your arm over the back of her chair, which will look to spectators as though it were round her neck; or, if she wears a low-necked dress, you can stand bending over her chair, looking down and praising the ring upon her finger, or the delicate whiteness of her hand. This will convince a lady that you have not only an inquiring mind, but that you also possess the natural instinct of a *well-bred* and *warm-hearted* gentleman.

Rule the Twenty-sixth

What is called *gassing* is a great card for a gentleman to play, especially with an accomplished and discriminating lady. Whenever he meets her, he must pretend that he has just come from a long and interesting conversation with Colonel this-one, and General that-one, or has just dined with Honorable Mister, or Governor so-and-so, and then speak of the great difficulty he had in tearing himself away from them. This will show her that he is conscious of possessing no merit of his own, to recommend him to her favor; which she will take as a pleasant and convincing proof of his modesty and humility, and which she will also charitably pass to his credit, against the lies which she well knows he is telling her.

Rule the Twenty-seventh

Always make yourself *comfortable* in the presence of a lady; which you may do, by sitting on the outer edge of your chair, and allowing your shoulders and body to fall backwards, while your legs are projecting forward into the middle of the room, and thrown apart like the divergent prongs of an immense pitch-fork. This is an elegant and tempting position. Then, in cold weather, you can sit down in her presence in your full winter rig, of overcoat, over-shoes, thick gloves and fur-cap, which will give you an air of great comfort, while it will, at the same time, be regarded as a sign of the most delicate respect for her presence. Or, you can accomplish the same desirable end, if the weather is hot, by going into her presence minus your suspenders and vest, with nothing on but your shirt, pantaloons, stockings and pumps. She will be sure to appreciate this delicate compliment to her presence, while she cannot fail to be struck with the justice and propriety of *puppies* achieving all the comforts they possibly can during *dog-days*.

Rule the Twenty-eighth

As *vanity* is considered one of the female virtues, you cannot do a better thing than to evince as much of it as possible. A convenient way to do this is to never forget *yourself* in the presence of a lady; that is, be more particular to render the occasion agreeable to yourself than you are to make it one of entire happiness to her; for this will show her that you *think too much of yourself* to descend to the small business of entertaining a woman. Talk, therefore, only of your own affairs. Be constantly adjusting your shirt-collar, or arranging your cravat, which will not only show that you are ambitious to look as handsome as possible, but it will be an employment for your hands, which might otherwise prove, in some way, an annoyance to her.

Rule the Twenty-ninth

There is no way in which you can be more serviceable and render yourself more agreeable to a lady than to bring her all the bad news you hear, especially if it relates to herself. All the disparaging things you hear said of her, you will, of course, take to her directly; which will cause her always to hail your coming with joy, while it proves, beyond a doubt, that you have been well-bred, and are a high-toned gentleman.

Rule the Thirtieth

If you suspect a lady to possess a considerable amount of strong good sense, and if you know her to have had some experience in the world, you may believe that you can easily win her confidence and respect, by *assuming* an extraordinary amount of piety, virtue, and respectability; which she well knows to be an old trick of nearly all young scape-graces, who have nothing *but pretension* in the great claims they make to morality. Therefore be easily shocked—be in constant alarm lest you should compromise yourself—put on pious airs; and the lady will give you credit for obeying the sublime injunction of the poet, who says:

> "Assume *a virtue—if you have it not.*"

Rule the Thirty-first

Always have some joke ready which is intended to be a hit at woman. For instance, if you see a lady eating a piece of tongue, you can remark that you are surprised to see her doing that, as you thought the ladies had already *tongue* enough. Some such original joke as this will impress a lady greatly in your favor, by convincing her that you are one of those commonplace, insipid creatures, whose intellect is down to the low level of woman's, and that you will not, therefore, be likely ever to startle and annoy her, by propositions or conversations beyond the reach of her comprehension.

Rule the Thirty-second

You will do well to follow the example of a great many gentlemen, and practise killing ways before the looking-glass, which will be quite sure to give you a style as charming and fascinating as the manners of a monkey, while it will flatter the vanity of any sensible woman to see what pains you take to render yourself so honorably agreeable to her sex.

Rule the Thirty-third

Always talk a little doubtingly of female virtue, for that will show that you are rigidly virtuous yourself, and that you associate chiefly with a class of women who cannot fail to be of great advantage to you in giving you proper, and sufficiently cautionary, ideas of the character of the sex.

Rule the Thirty-Fourth

Pretend that you are perfectly invulnerable to all the charms of woman, which will convince her that you are the most vulnerable and susceptible creature alive, and that you are always making love to every pretty woman you see, married or single. This will show that your heart is as tender as though it were *rotten*, and that you would, therefore, make a most excellent and desirable husband.

Rule the Thirty-Fifth

Also, talk perpetually of your great caution as to what women you associate with. The louder your professions in this matter, the more you will convince a sensible lady that you would make love even to your washer-woman, without regard to color, and that your wife, therefore, may reasonably expect to be relieved of a great deal of the persecution of a husband's affections.

Rule the Thirty-sixth

Always complain that your lady acquaintances are too numerous, and absorb too much of your time, which will convince a discerning woman that you have not a single respectable female acquaintance except herself, and that she, therefore, has you all to herself, including all your pretensions and lies.

Rule the Thirty-seventh

If there is a beautiful married lady in your neighborhood, you will, of course, try to flirt with her; and, as a preparatory step, you will cultivate the confidence and friendship of her husband, which is a most direct road to the affections of the wife; for it will thoroughly apprise her of your designs, and then nothing will delight her more than to witness your efforts to impose upon her husband. If she is really worth flirting with, your success will be certain, and you will have the pleasure of being laughed at by those adroit rascals who always avoid the friendship and even the acquaintance of a man, with whose wife they desire to flirt.

Rule the Thirty-eighth

It is a masterly stroke of policy of some young men to be always railing at matrimony—an example I advise you, by all means, to copy, for it will give you an opportunity of courting every pretty woman who comes in your way, without being suspected of any but the most unselfish and honorable intentions. A man who despises matrimony, and who avows his determination never to marry, has also a *carte blanche* to the home of every young lady; for the parents know that there is no danger that he will ever steal away their daughter permanently in marriage, his object being only a temporary courtship.

Rule the Thirty-ninth

There is an insipid tribe of triflers, called "danglers," with whom women are very fond of diverting themselves in mock flirtations, when they have nothing better to do. They regard them as a class of beings beneath their monkeys, parrots, and lap-dogs; but, possessing the form, and, in some degree, the attributes of a man, they use them for pastime, and to practise themselves in the pleasant art of flirting. It will cost you but little pains to become one of these useful and happy beings.

Rule the Fortieth

If you have made up your mind to strike a woman quite *dead in love* with you, fix your eyes amorously upon hers, and gaze fixedly and burningly into them, as though you were mesmerizing her. If you perceive that it is with difficulty she keeps from laughing in your face, or, if she turns away her face in scorn, as though she felt insulted, you must, by no means, relax your gaze, for these are clear signs that you are having your effect upon her. And if she sends for her father, or brother, to kick you out of the house, you may know that it is because she dare not longer trust herself in your fascinating presence.

Rule the Forty-first

What is called *attitudinizing* is a great game to play upon an intelligent and sensible woman—that is, to throw your body into a series of graceful pictures, or fascinating attitudes, which you must study before a mirror; and, as a lady will readily detect your skill and practice, she will at once bite at so tempting a bait, and set herself to win your heart, as sincerely as a spider spins a fine web to catch a fly, for she knows that all such insects are easily caught, and easily bled.

Rule the Forty-second

If you perceive that a lady is decidedly averse to receiving you, and actually flies from your presence, you should perpetually throw yourself under her nose, on the same principle that a horse is made to smell of a wheel-barrow to keep him from taking fright at such an ugly machine.

Rule the Forty-third

Or, if a lady begins to show evident signs of weariness at your frequent calls, by all means double your attentions— call oftener, and stay longer, until you make yourself a fixture in her presence, like a dummy in the door-way of a haberdasher. This will soon do the business for you, and leave no possible grounds to doubt as to your real position in her affections.

Rule the Forty-fourth

If a lady condescends to treat you with a little familiarity, you must instantly take advantage of it, and make your-self as familiar and as agreeable as possible, which you may do by some trick as sticking your segar almost into her eyes, to light it, or taking her finger to brush the ashes from the end of it; and if she should ask you why you do not use your own finger, you can reply by making a double nose, and say "no you don't," which will strike her with admiration both for your wit and familiar good breeding.

Rule the Forty-fifth

Nothing makes a gentleman appear to so great advantage as to be good at "small talk," that is, to be able to prattle away for hours without saying anything. If you have not this fascinating gift of gab yourself, you will do well to take along some such help as Harper's monthly picture-book, so that you can amuse the lady by studying the jokes to find out where the laughs come in. If you should be unable to find any, you can make a joke yourself, by pulling the lady's nose, and exclaiming "not as you nose-on;" and then, by laughing as loud as you can scream, you will prove that your own unaided wit and genius have found a joke.

Rule the Forty-sixth

It is a delightful and sprightly species of wit, called *big talk*, which accomplished gentlemen sometimes indulge in to entertain ladies by descriptions of mock adventures, such as riding an earthquake to water, drinking out of the milky-way, cutting a piece off of the spectre of the Brocken for a night-cap, catching a comet by the tail, or hunting for a calf's head in the cell of a moon beam. If, after you have delivered yourself of this matchless piece of sense and humor, the lady gravely asks if you had any difficulty in finding a *calf's head*, you may know that she fully appreciates your genius, and that you have made an immense hit.

Rule the Forty-seventh

I advise you to study to perform a few pleasing and charming tricks in every lady's presence, such as snatch-ing her pocket-handkerchief out of her lap and throwing it upon the floor, and violently stamping upon it; and when she asks, with terror, what you are doing, reply that you are killing a *wiper*. Or you can open the door on a winter's night, and then astonish and delight her by asking if there are any *pickles in it?* and when she asks what you mean, reply, "nothing, only I see it is *a-jar*." A few such tricks as these will convince a lady that you would be as amusing in a house as a monkey, and therefore would be a great prize as a husband.

Rule the Forty-eighth

If you intend to call on a lady in the evening, do not neglect to drink liquor several times, and several kinds of it, during the day, for this will give spirit to your conversation, while it will enable you to perfume her whole house with a fragrance which can be equalled only by a scent that has now become very rare, in consequence of the scarcity of the animal that produces it.

Rule the Forty-ninth

Giggle and laugh perpetually—make fun, even of serious things; for that will show that your heart is as light as your head, and that grief is as great a stranger to the one as sense to the other.

Rule the Fiftieth

If you have not the natural sprightliness and playfulness to enable you to take advantage of these rules, take the other tack, and be as surly as possible—that is, if you cannot be a *puppy* and frisk and bark, be an old dog and growl.

INDEX

Madame Lola Montez

was born in 1818 in Limerick, the daughter of an army officer, and christened Maria Dolores Eliza Rosana Gilbert. At the age of seventeen she eloped in order to prevent her mother from marrying her to a titled octogenarian residing in India. The marriage did not last long, and to support herself she became a Spanish dancer, using the name of Lola Montez. Her specialty was a dance in which she pretended to have spiders in her petticoats and had to shake them out.

She was a sensational success in Europe, due primarily to her great beauty and charm. She became the friend of Tsar Nicholas I, Franz Liszt, Balzac, and Alexandre Dumas, who said, "In her was mind and heart enough for a dozen kings." In Paris, she was the cause of a duel in which one of her lovers was killed, and she left France for Vienna. There she met and captivated Ludwig I of Bavaria, who made her Countess of Landsfeld and Baroness Rosenthal. For a time she wielded tremendous power and influence in Germany, but Ludwig was forced to abdicate in 1848, and she had to flee.

A few years later she came to New York, and was the companion of Walt Whitman, Willian Dean Howells, and Commodore Vanderbilt. She moved west, married, and settled for a while on a ranch in California, where, according to neighbors, she kept exotic animals, "wore men's clothes, and horeswhipped editors." Lola Montez gave lectures on fashion, beauty, and gallantry, and wrote her autobiography. She eventually returned to New York, where, as Eliza Gilbert, she worked to save wayward women. She died in 1861, a religious recluse, and is buried in Greenwood Cemetery in Brooklyn.